THE PLANT BASED HIGH PROTEIN COOKBOOK

Increase your energy with quick and easy vegan recipes. A nutrition guide for a healthy lifestyle. Improve your workout, grow your muscle & get in shape.

Jules Whole

Table of Contents

Chapter 9.   Low Calories Recipes 237

Introduction

What is a plant-based diet?

As you might or might not understand, healthy proteins are made up of amino acids, called the "structure blocks" of life. Healthy protein assists create enzymes, hormonal agents, antibodies, and creating brand-new cells. The human body can make 9 of the 22 amino acids that make up healthy proteins.

Arginine

Identified as a semi-essential or "conditionally" necessary amino acid, they rely on the developing phase and health and wellness condition of the person. It can be found in: almonds, beetroots, brazil nuts, buckwheat, carrots, cashews, celery, chickpeas, coconut, cucumbers, flaxseed, garlic, green veggies, hazelnuts, kidney beans, leeks, lentil, lettuce, dietary yeast, onion, parsnips, pecans, want nuts, potatoes, pumpkin seeds, radishes, sesame seeds, sprouts, sunflower seeds, and walnuts.

Histidine

Particularly required throughout early stages for the correct development and growth – it used to be thought to be just important for infants, yet, it is currently recognized to be necessary for grownups.

It can be found in apples, bananas, beans, beetroots, buckwheat, carrots, melon, cauliflower, celery, citrus fruits, cucumber, dandelion, endive, garlic, eco-friendlies, beans, mushrooms, pomegranates, radish, rice, algae, sesame, spirulina, spinach, and turnip.

Isoleucine

Essential for muscle mass upkeep, manufacturing, and healing – particularly post-workout. It is associated with hemoglobin development, the management of blood sugar levels, embolism's development, and power.

It can be found in almonds, avocados, cashews, chickpeas, coconut, lentils, olives, papaya, algae, and most seeds like sunflower.

Leucine

Necessary for development hormonal agent manufacturing, cell manufacturing, and repair service, it stops muscle mass loss. It is used when dealing with problems such as parkinson's condition.

It can be found in almonds, asparagus, avocados, chickpeas, coconut, lentils, oats, olives, papayas, rice, sunflower seeds, and walnuts.

Lysine

Great for calcium absorption, bone growth, nitrogen upkeep, cell repair work, hormonal agent manufacturing, antibody manufacturing.

It can be found in amaranth, apples, apricots, beans, beetroots, carrots, celery, cucumber, dandelion eco-friendlies, grapes, papayas, parsley, pears, peas, spinach, and turnip eco-friendlies.

Methionine

It is described as the "cleaner" – essential for fat emulsification, food digestion, anti-oxidant (cancer cells avoidance), arterial plaque avoidance (heart wellness), and heavy metal elimination.

It can be found in black beans, brazil nuts, cashews, kidney beans, oats, sesame seeds, spirulina, spinach, sunflower seeds, and watercress.

Phenylalanine

A forerunner for tyrosine and the indicating particles of dopamine, norepinephrine (noradrenaline), and epinephrine (adrenaline), in addition, a forerunner to the skin pigment: melanin. Sustains understanding and memory, mind procedures, and altitude perception.

It can be found in apples, beetroots, carrots, cashews, flaxseed, hazelnuts, dietary yeast, parsley, pineapples, pumpkin seeds, sesame seeds, sunflower seeds, spinach, and tomatoes.

Threonine

Screens physical healthy proteins for their preservation or reuse.

It can be found in almonds, beans, carrots, celery, chickpeas, collards, flaxseed, eco-friendlies, green leafy veggies, kale, lentils, lima beans, nori, nuts, papayas, sesame seeds, sunflower seeds, and walnuts.

Tryptophan

It is required for niacin and serotonin manufacturing, discomfort perception, and monitoring of the rest of the body.

It can be found in brussels sprouts, carrots, celery, chives, dandelion eco-friendlies, endive, fennel, dietary yeast, pumpkin seeds, sesame seeds, break beans, spinach, sunflower seeds, walnuts, and turnips.

Valine

Aids muscular tissue manufacturing, healing, strength, endurance - balance nitrogen degrees, and it is utilized in the therapy of alcohol-related mental retardation.

It can be found in apples, almonds, bananas, beetroots, broccoli, carrots, celery, dandelion environment-friendlies, lettuce, dietary yeast, okra, parsley, parsnips, pomegranates, potatoes, squash, turnips, and tomatoes.

Within the world of plant-based diet regimens, there are a lot of different kinds. A vegetarian diet plan excludes meat (fowl, beef, pork, and all the others), fish and, shellfish. It, however, typically includes eggs and milk and milk-derived products (the term "lacto-ovo vegetarian" uses below). A "pescatarian" diet plan refers to a plant-based diet plan that additionally includes fish and/or fish and shellfish, however, no meat is present.

Benefits of Vegan Diet

There are several benefits to a vegan diet, especially when it comes to nutrition. You will consume a lot of nutrients and far less saturated fats. As great as this sounds, it can be challenging for someone to give up their animal-based foods because they need to find alternative sources of their protein, vitamins, minerals, iron, and non-saturated fats. If they don't plan their new diet carefully, it could potentially cause them to face certain health risks.

The people who go on a vegan diet may do so for more than just health reasons. They may be taking a stand to promote environmental protection and stopping animal cruelty.

Nutritional benefits:

• Reduced saturated fats: vegan diet has less saturated fats which improve health, especially when it comes to coronary diseases

• More energy: more carbs in a plant-based diet provide energy to the body , fiber: high fiber vegan diet leads to healthier bowel movement and help in fighting against colon cancer

• Anti-oxidants: vegetables and fruits are rich in antioxidants that protect the body from some types of cancer

• Vitamins: vitamins boost the immune system, heals wounds faster and benefit skin, eyes, brain, and heart.

Disease prevention:

• Cardiovascular disease: improve cardiovascular health and prevent heart attack and stroke

• Cholesterol: eliminating animal foods means eliminating dietary cholesterol which improves heart health

• Blood pressure: vegan diet is rich in whole foods which is beneficial in lowering high blood pressure

- Cancer: switching to a vegan diet reversed many illnesses like reducing chances of prostate cancer, colon cancer, and breast cancer
- Arthritis: plant-based diet is very promising for improving health in individuals suffering from arthritis

Physical benefits

- Body mass index (bmi): diet without meats lowers bmi which is an indicator of healthy weight loss
- Weight loss: vegan diet eliminates unhealthy foods that tend to cause weight gain
- Healthy skin: vitamins and other essential nutrients from vegetables makes skin healthy, so vegans have good healthy skin
- Longer life: vegan lives three to six years longer than people who don't follow a vegan or vegetarian lifestyle
- Body odor: eliminating meat and dairy product from diet reduce body odor, and body smells better
- Hairs and nails: individuals who follow a vegan diet have strong hairs and healthier nails
- Migraines and allergies: vegan diet is a relief from migraines and reduces allergy symptoms, runny nose, and congestion.

Bodybuilding

The ideal muscle construction diet drinks

Apart from getting protein from foods, you might even get it out of protein shakes. Shakes are a superior diet in assisting to gain muscle. Shakes are easy to create and may be employed by the body contractors that have many responsibilities and they lack time to prepare plant-based foods which have high protein content. The right time to eat the protein shakes is through the daytime hours before a workout.

A healthful balanced vegetarian diet program takes consideration and research. If you make the choice to be a vegetarian, you'll end up confronted with many options. There are several distinct types of vegetarian diets. Some include eggs and milk, others have one or another contained, and others include some animal products on occasion. Then you will find the vegans who have a rigorous plant-based diet with no dairy, no eggs, and no animal products. You'll also discover that many vegans are cautious to not wear, or make use of any products that are related to animals such as gelatin or honey. Vegans are usually quite conscious of their ethical treatment of animals.

When you choose a balanced vegetarian diet plan, you'll have to know about each the minerals and vitamins you will have to supplement to get adequate nutrition in your diet on a daily basis. There are a few vitamins and minerals which are lacking in a conventional plant-based diet such as iron, zinc, magnesium, vitamin b-12, vitamin d, vitamin and protein. A few of the vitamins and minerals are located in a daily multivitamin, or at different nutritional supplements. Listed here are a few of the advantages and foods to look for in a healthful vegetarian diet program.

Iron is an essential nutrient because it carries oxygen from the blood. Since iron is most frequently seen in a nonvegetarian diet, vegetarians and vegans will need to locate excellent sources of iron in many different foods. Such foods comprise sea vegetables such as wakame, and nori, iron fortified cereals, legumes, tofu, and dried fruits.

Zinc is a mineral that's usually found in milk products. Vegetarians can get this nutrient in foods such as soy products, and quite a few cereals.

Calcium strengthens bones and teeth, and may also be found chiefly in milk product. You could even locate calcium in certain cereals, tofu, soy milk, and orange juice with additional calcium.

Vitamin b-12 is vital for blood formation and cell division. It can typically be seen in animal products such as eggs and milk, and vegetarians may discover this vitamin foods such as fortified cereals and soy milk. Vitamin d is a vitamin frequently found in milk products. Everybody may benefit from vitamin d to keep them healthy and strong. It's also proven to increase the mood. It may be located in exposure to sunlight, mushrooms, and in fortified cereals.

Protein is essential for maintaining muscle and bone mass. It's generally seen in animal products, nevertheless vegetarians may get sufficient protein via soy based products, legumes, tofu, peanut butter, and nuts.

Understanding what foods to eat in a healthier balanced vegetarian diet is essential for staying healthy and vital. You are going to want to perform the study before starting any new diet program. As soon as you choose a balanced vegetarian diet program, you may wish to educate yourself, and decide which diet plan is ideal for you. Eating a wide variety of foods is better, and in the event you're able to supplement your diet with essential minerals and vitamins, you'll be ahead of the match.

What protein can do to help your body

- Eating protein is able to help you keep a healthful weight. Should you increase muscle mass, then the accession of the exceptionally metabolic tissue can assist with weight control.

- You do not have to consume meat for this to be authentic. Tofu can help, so can protein powders from plant resources: veggies, hemp or brown rice, such as.

- Protein is made from amino acids. The amino acids make enzymes to break down any protein that you consume.

- Protein is used for generation of blood cells, which transport nearly every material within the body.

- Protein reinforces muscle structure and can be utilized for protective structuring in the skin, white blood cells, red blood cells, and even much more.

- Protein is utilized to fix and replace muscle, tendons and other tissues, especially after instruction, in addition to in mucus production.

- Muscle protein may be utilized as a fuel supply. It's actually the 2nd biggest source of stored fuel in your system.

- Protein is utilized to create hormones.

- Protein is utilized to create hormones and other brain chemicals.
- Protein plays a significant part in the immune system, which can not work without it.

The all-important immune system

We in turn could not operate with no immune system. It protects against, and assists in healing from, germs, disease and disease. The immune system also manages healing from wounds, injury, burns, and operation.

Another significant facet of immune function is recovery from workouts.

The immune system is much too complicated to cover in a brief article on overall uses of nourishment. 1 cool truth, however, involves the adaptive immune system (ais). The ais is made from protein cells known as b-lymphocytes, generated in bone marrow and published since"scanner proteins" b-lymphocytes scan the entire body searching for invading bodies. As soon as they identify the proper"lock and key"they eliminate the invading body.

Protein also provides the fuel the immune system operates : l-glutamine. Glutamine is an amino acid and discovered chiefly in foods. It's also found in plant foods at reduced amounts.

Glutamine's other valuable functions contain muscle maintenance, intestinal and digestive health, glutathione (antioxidant) manufacturing, ph balance, and blood vessel health.

Foods comprising l-glutamine contain sea foods, fish (saltwater fish possess significantly more glutamine than freshwater), mussel, fish, fish, grass-fed steak, poultry, lamb, bone broth. Milk and milk products (yogurt, ricotta cheese) provide glutamine, too. Other animal proteins using high glutamine content are organ meats, especially liver.

Plant sources of glutamine contain raw red cabbage, chickpeas, lentils, legumes, asparagus, nuts, parsley, spinach, collard greens, spinach, cilantro, radish greens, along with an assortment of fruits.

Chapter 1. Breakfast

Spinach and Berries Salad

Preparation time: 5 minutes

Cooking time: 0 minutes

Servings: 4

Ingredients:

1 cup baby spinach

1 cup blackberries

1 cup blueberries

1 tablespoon avocado oil

1 tablespoon balsamic vinegar

1 tablespoon parsley, chopped

½ cup pine nuts, chopped

Salt and black pepper to the taste

Directions:

In a salad bowl, combine the spinach with the berries and the other ingredients, toss and serve for breakfast.

Nutrition: calories 158, fat 12.4, fiber 3.8, carbs 11.5, protein 3.4

Cauliflower hash

Preparation time: 10 minutes

Cooking time: 15 minutes

Servings: 4

Ingredients:

2 cups cauliflower florets, roughly chopped

½ teaspoon basil, dried

1 teaspoon sage, dried

2 spring onions, chopped

1 tablespoon avocado oil

½ cup coconut cream

½ teaspoon sweet paprika

Salt and black pepper to the taste

1 tablespoon cilantro, chopped

Directions:

Heat up a pan with the oil over medium heat, add the onions and sauté for 5 minutes.

Add the cauliflower and the other ingredients, toss, cook everything for 10 minutes more, divide between plates and serve for breakfast.

Nutrition: calories 90, fat 7.7, fiber 2.4, carbs 5.3, protein 1.9

Spinach and Green Beans Casserole

Preparation time: 10 minutes

Cooking time: 40 minutes

Servings: 4

Ingredients:

1 pound green beans, trimmed and halved

4 scallions, chopped

1 tablespoon coconut oil, melted

1 cup baby spinach

2 tablespoons flaxseed mixed with 3 tablespoons water

½ cup cashew cheese, grated

Salt and black pepper to the taste

½ teaspoon thyme, chopped

Directions:

Heat up a pan with the oil over medium heat, add the scallions and sauté for 5 minutes.

Add the green beans and the other ingredients except the cheese, stir and cook for 5 minutes more.

Sprinkle the cheese on top and bake the mix at 390 degrees f for 30 minutes.

Divide the mix between plates and serve.

Nutrition: calories 273, fat 13.7, fiber 0.2, carbs 2.2, protein 1.5

Spiced Zucchini and Eggplant Bowls

Preparation time: 10 minutes

Cooking time: 15 minutes

Servings: 4

Ingredients:

1 tablespoon olive oil

4 scallions, chopped

2 zucchinis, cubed

1 eggplants, cubed

1 tablespoon cilantro, chopped

1 teaspoon rosemary, dried

1 teaspoon allspice, ground

1 teaspoon nutmeg, ground

¼ cup coconut cream

Salt and black pepper to the taste

1 tablespoons chives, chopped

Directions:

Heat up a pan with the oil over medium heat, add the scallions, allspice and the nutmeg and sauté for 5 minutes.

Add the zucchini is, eggplant and the other ingredients, toss, cook over medium heat for 10 minutes, divide into bowls and serve for breakfast,

Nutrition: calories 242, fat 6.4, fiber 2, carbs 10, protein 2

Spinach and Berries Salad

Preparation time: 5 minutes

Cooking time: 0 minutes

Servings: 4

Ingredients:

1 cup baby spinach

1 cup blackberries

1 cup blueberries

1 tablespoon avocado oil

1 tablespoon balsamic vinegar

1 tablespoon parsley, chopped

½ cup pine nuts, chopped

Salt and black pepper to the taste

Directions:

In a salad bowl, combine the spinach with the berries and the other ingredients, toss and serve for breakfast.

Nutrition: calories 158, fat 12.4, fiber 3.8, carbs 11.5, protein 3.4

Cauliflower hash

Preparation time: 10 minutes

Cooking time: 15 minutes

Servings: 4

Ingredients:

2 cups cauliflower florets, roughly chopped

½ teaspoon basil, dried

1 teaspoon sage, dried

2 spring onions, chopped

1 tablespoon avocado oil

½ cup coconut cream

½ teaspoon sweet paprika

Salt and black pepper to the taste

1 tablespoon cilantro, chopped

Directions:

Heat up a pan with the oil over medium heat, add the onions and sauté for 5 minutes.

Add the cauliflower and the other ingredients, toss, cook everything for 10 minutes more, divide between plates and serve for breakfast.

Nutrition: calories 90, fat 7.7, fiber 2.4, carbs 5.3, protein 1.9

Spinach and Green Beans Casserole

Preparation time: 10 minutes

Cooking time: 40 minutes

Servings: 4

Ingredients:

1 pound green beans, trimmed and halved

4 scallions, chopped

1 tablespoon coconut oil, melted

1 cup baby spinach

2 tablespoons flaxseed mixed with 3 tablespoons water

½ cup cashew cheese, grated

Salt and black pepper to the taste

½ teaspoon thyme, chopped

Directions:

Heat up a pan with the oil over medium heat, add the scallions and sauté for 5 minutes.

Add the green beans and the other ingredients except the cheese, stir and cook for 5 minutes more.

Sprinkle the cheese on top and bake the mix at 390 degrees f for 30 minutes.

Divide the mix between plates and serve.

Nutrition: calories 273, fat 13.7, fiber 0.2, carbs 2.2, protein 1.5

Spiced Zucchini and Eggplant Bowls

Preparation time: 10 minutes

Cooking time: 15 minutes

Servings: 4

Ingredients:

1 tablespoon olive oil

4 scallions, chopped

2 zucchinis, cubed

1 eggplants, cubed

1 tablespoon cilantro, chopped

1 teaspoon rosemary, dried

1 teaspoon allspice, ground

1 teaspoon nutmeg, ground

¼ cup coconut cream

Salt and black pepper to the taste

1 tablespoons chives, chopped

Directions:

Heat up a pan with the oil over medium heat, add the scallions, allspice and the nutmeg and sauté for 5 minutes.

Add the zucchini is, eggplant and the other ingredients, toss, cook over medium heat for 10 minutes, divide into bowls and serve for breakfast,

Nutrition: calories 242, fat 6.4, fiber 2, carbs 10, protein 2

Zucchini muffins

Preparation time: 5 minutes

Cooking time: 30 minutes

Servings: 6

Ingredients:

4 scallions, chopped

1 tablespoon olive oil

2 zucchinis, chopped

1 yellow bell pepper, chopped

Salt and black pepper to the taste

2 tablespoons flaxseed mixed with 3 tablespoons water

1 cup almond flour

1 cup almond milk

1 teaspoon baking powder

2 tablespoons chives, chopped

Directions:

Heat up a pan with the oil over medium heat, add the scallions, zucchini is and the bell pepper and sauté for 5 minutes.

In a bowl, combine the scallions mix with the rest of the ingredients, stir well, divide into a muffin tray and bake at 390 degrees f for 25 minutes.

Divide the muffins between plates and serve them for breakfast.

Nutrition: calories 258, fat 21.8, fiber 4.9, carbs 11.9, protein 6.6

Berry and Dates Oatmeal

Preparation time: 5 minutes

Cooking time: 0 minutes

Servings: 2

Ingredients:

½ cup coconut flesh, unsweetened and shredded

1 cup coconut milk

¼ cup dates, chopped

1 teaspoon vanilla extract

1 tablespoon stevia

1 cup berries, mashed

Directions:

In a bowl, combine the coconut flesh with the coconut milk, the dates and the other ingredients, whisk well, divide into 2 bowls and serve.

Nutrition: calories 572, fat 47.2, fiber 11.5, carbs 38.8, protein 5.8

Tomato oatmeal

Preparation time: 5 minutes

Cooking time: 20 minutes

Servings: 4

Ingredients:

3 cups water

1 cup coconut milk

1 tablespoon avocado oil

1 cup coconut flesh, unsweetened and shredded

¼ cup cherry tomatoes, chopped

A pinch of red pepper flakes

1 teaspoon chili powder

Directions:

Meanwhile, heat up a pan with the oil over medium-high heat, add the tomatoes, chili powder and pepper flakes and sauté for 5 minutes

Add the coconut and sauté for 5 minutes more.

Add the remaining ingredients, toss, bring to a simmer, cook over medium heat fro 10 minutes more, divide into bowls and serve for breakfast.

Nutrition: calories 170, fat 17.8, fiber 1.5, carbs 3.8, protein 1.5

Mushroom muffins

Preparation time: 10 minutes

Cooking time: 30 minutes

Servings: 8

Ingredients:

1 cup cauliflower rice

2 tablespoons flaxseed mixed with 3 tablespoons water

Salt and black pepper to the taste

1 cup cashew cheese, grated

4 scallions, chopped

1 red bell pepper chopped

1 cup white mushrooms, sliced

Cooking spray

Directions:

In a bowl, combine the cauliflower rice with the flaxseed mix, scallions and the other ingredients, and whisk well.

Grease a muffin pan with the cooking spray, divide the mushrooms mix, bake at 350 degrees f for 30 minutes and serve for breakfast.

Nutrition: calories 123, fat 5.6, fiber 1.3, carbs 10.8, protein 7.5

Soy yogurt morning shake

Preparation time: 5 minutes

cooking time: 14 hours, Servings: 4

Ingredients:

For the shake:

1 (32 oz) vegan soy milk

2 tbsp plain vegan yogurt

2 frozen bananas, peeled

1 (8 oz) canned apricots, drained

For topping:

1 apricot, pitted and chopped

Chia seeds

Chopped pistachios

Directions:

Share the soy-milk into two large mason jars and add a tablespoon of vegan yogurt each. Close the jars with the covers and place both in the pot.

Close the pot's lid, secure the pressure valve, and select Yogurt mode. Set the timer for 14 hours. When ready, perform a quick pressure release.

In a blender, add the yogurt, bananas, and apricots. Process the ingredients until smooth and divide into breakfast glasses. Top with apricots, chia seeds, and pistachios.

Nutrition:

Calories 189, carbohydrates 31.2 g, fats 5.5 g, protein 5.1 g

Chapter 2. Lunch

Avocado, Spinach and Kale Soup

Preparation time: 10 minutes

Cooking time: 0 minutes

Servings: 4

Ingredients:

2 avocados, pitted, peeled and cut in halves

4 cups vegetable stock

2 tablespoons cilantro, chopped

Juice of 1 lime

1 teaspoon rosemary, dried

½ cup spinach leaves

½ cup kale, torn

Salt and black pepper to the taste

Directions:

In a blender, combine the avocados with the stock and the other ingredients, pulse well, divide into bowls and serve for lunch.

Nutrition: calories 300, fat 23, fiber 5, carbs 6, protein 7

Curry spinach soup

Preparation time: 10 minutes

Cooking time: 0 minutes

Servings: 4

Ingredients:

1 cup almond milk

1 tablespoon green curry paste

1 pound spinach leaves

1 tablespoon cilantro, chopped

Salt and black pepper to the taste

4 cups veggie stock

1 tablespoon cilantro, chopped

Directions:

In your blender, combine the almond milk with the curry paste and the other ingredients, pulse well, divide into bowls and serve for lunch.

Nutrition: calories 240, fat 4, fiber 2, carbs 6, protein 2

Arugula and Artichokes Bowls

Preparation time: 5 minutes

Cooking time: 0 minutes

Servings: 4

Ingredients:

2 cups baby arugula

¼ cup walnuts, chopped

1 cup canned artichoke hearts, drained and quartered

1 tablespoon balsamic vinegar

2 tablespoons cilantro, chopped

2 tablespoons olive oil

Salt and black pepper to the taste

1 tablespoon lemon juice

Directions:

In a bowl, combine the artichokes with the arugula, walnuts and the other ingredients, toss, divide into smaller bowls and serve for lunch.

Nutrition: calories 200, fat 2, fiber 1, carbs 5, protein 7

Minty arugula soup

Preparation time: 5 minutes

Cooking time: 10 minutes

Servings: 4

Ingredients:

3 scallions, chopped

1 tablespoon olive oil

½ Cup coconut milk

2 cups baby arugula

2 tablespoons mint, chopped

6 cups vegetable stock

2 tablespoons chives, chopped

Salt and black pepper to the taste

Directions:

Heat up a pot with the oil over medium high heat, add the scallions and sauté for 2 minutes.

Add the rest of the ingredients, toss, bring to a simmer and cook over medium heat for 8 minutes more.

Divide the soup into bowls and serve.

Nutrition: calories 200, fat 4, fiber 2, carbs 6, protein 10

Spinach and Broccoli Soup

Preparation time: 10 minutes

Cooking time: 20 minutes

Servings: 4

Ingredients:

3 shallots, chopped

1 tablespoon olive oil

2 garlic cloves, minced

½ pound broccoli florets

½ pound baby spinach

Salt and black pepper to the taste

4 cups veggie stock

1 teaspoon turmeric powder

1 tablespoon lime juice

Directions:

Heat up a pot with the oil over medium high heat, add the shallots and the garlic and sauté for 5 minutes.

Add the broccoli, spinach and the other ingredients, toss, bring to a simmer and cook over medium heat for 15 minutes.

Ladle into soup bowls and serve.

Nutrition: calories 150, fat 3, fiber 1, carbs 3, protein 7

Coconut zucchini cream

Preparation time: 10 minutes

Cooking time: 25 minutes

Servings: 4

Ingredients:

1 pound zucchinis, roughly chopped

2 tablespoons avocado oil

4 scallions, chopped

Salt and black pepper to the taste

6 cups veggie stock

1 teaspoon basil, dried

1 teaspoon cumin, ground

3 garlic cloves, minced

¾ cup coconut cream

1 tablespoon dill, chopped

Directions:

Heat up a pot with the oil over medium high heat, add the scallions and the garlic and sauté for 5 minutes.

Add the rest of the ingredients, stir, bring to a simmer and cook over medium heat for 20 minutes more.

Blend the soup using an immersion blender, ladle into bowls and serve.

Nutrition: calories 160, fat 4, fiber 2, carbs 4, protein 8

Zucchini and Cauliflower Soup

Preparation time: 10 minutes

Cooking time: 25 minutes

Servings: 4

Ingredients:

4 scallions, chopped

1 teaspoon ginger, grated

2 tablespoons olive oil

1 pound zucchinis, sliced

2 cups cauliflower florets

Salt and black pepper to the taste

6 cups veggie stock

1 garlic clove, minced

1 tablespoon lemon juice

1 cup coconut cream

Directions:

Heat up a pot with the oil over medium heat, add the scallions, ginger and the garlic and sauté for 5 minutes. Add the rest of the ingredients, bring to a simmer and cook over medium heat for 20 minutes.

Blend everything using an immersion blender, ladle into soup bowls and serve.

Nutrition: calories 154, fat 12, fiber 3, carbs 5, protein 4

Chard soup

Preparation time: 10 minutes

Cooking time: 25 minutes

Servings: 4

Ingredients:

1 pound Swiss chard, chopped

½ cup shallots, chopped

1 tablespoon avocado oil

1 teaspoon cumin, ground

1 teaspoon rosemary, dried

1 teaspoon basil, dried

2 garlic cloves, minced

Salt and black pepper to the taste

6 cups vegetable stock

1 tablespoon tomato passata

1 tablespoon cilantro, chopped

Directions:

Heat up a pan with the oil over medium heat, add the shallots and the garlic and sauté for 5 minutes.

Add the swiss chard and the other ingredients, toss, bring to a simmer and cook over medium heat for 20 minutes more.

Divide the soup into bowls and serve.

Nutrition: calories 232, fat 23, fiber 3, carbs 4, protein 3

Avocado, Pine Nuts and Chard Salad

Preparation time: 5 minutes

Cooking time: 15 minutes

Servings: 4

Ingredients:

1 pound swiss chard, roughly chopped

2 tablespoons olive oil

1 avocado, peeled, pitted and roughly cubed

2 spring onions, chopped

¼ Cup pine nuts, toasted

1 tablespoon balsamic vinegar

Salt and black pepper to the taste

Directions:

Heat up a pan with the oil over medium heat, add the spring onions, pine nuts and the chard, stir and sauté for 5 minutes.

Add the vinegar and the other ingredients, toss, cook over medium heat for 10 minutes more, divide into bowls and serve for lunch.

Nutrition: calories 120, fat 2, fiber 1, carbs 4, protein 8

Grapes, Avocado and Spinach Salad

Preparation time: 10 minutes

Cooking time: 0 minutes

Servings: 4

Ingredients:

1 cup green grapes, halved

2 cups baby spinach

1 avocado, pitted, peeled and cubed

Salt and black pepper to the taste

2 tablespoons olive oil

1 tablespoon thyme, chopped

1 tablespoon rosemary, chopped

1 tablespoon lime juice

1 garlic clove, minced

Directions:

In a salad bowl, combine the grapes with the spinach and the other ingredients, toss, and serve for lunch.

Nutrition: calories 190, fat 17.1, fiber 4.6, carbs 10.9, protein 1.7

Greens and Olives Pan

Preparation time: 10 minutes

Cooking time: 15 minutes

Servings: 4

Ingredients:

4 spring onions, chopped

2 tablespoons olive oil

½ cup green olives, pitted and halved

¼ cup pine nuts, toasted

1 tablespoon balsamic vinegar

2 cups baby spinach

1 cup baby arugula

1 cup asparagus, trimmed, blanched and halved

Salt and black pepper to the taste

Directions:

Heat up a pan with the oil over medium high heat, add the spring onions and the asparagus and sauté for 5 minutes.

Add the olives, spinach and the other ingredients, toss, cook over medium heat for 10 minutes, divide between plates and serve for lunch.

Nutrition: calories 136, fat 13.1, fiber 1.9, carbs 4.4, protein 2.8

Mushrooms and Chard Soup

Preparation time: 10 minutes

Cooking time: 30 minutes

Servings: 4

Ingredients:

3 cups Swiss chard, chopped

6 cups vegetable stock

1 cup mushrooms, sliced

2 garlic cloves, minced

1 tablespoon olive oil

2 scallions, chopped

2 tablespoons balsamic vinegar

¼ cup basil, chopped

Salt and black pepper to the taste

1 tablespoon cilantro, chopped

Directions:

Heat up a pot with the oil over medium high heat, add the scallions and the garlic and sauté for 5 minutes.

Add the mushrooms and sauté for another 5 minutes.

Add the rest of the ingredients, toss, bring to a simmer and cook over medium heat for 20 minutes more.

Ladle the soup into bowls and serve.

Nutrition: calories 140, fat 4, fiber 2, carbs 4, protein 8

Tomato, Green Beans and Chard Soup

Preparation time: 10 minutes

Cooking time: 35 minutes

Servings: 4

Ingredients:

2 scallions, chopped

1 cup swiss chard, chopped

1 tablespoon olive oil

1 red bell pepper, chopped

Salt and black pepper to the taste

1 cup tomatoes, cubed

1 cup green beans, chopped

6 cups vegetable stock

2 tablespoons tomato passata

2 garlic cloves, minced

2 teaspoons thyme, chopped

½ Teaspoon red pepper flakes

Directions:

Heat up a pot with the oil over medium heat, add the scallions, garlic and the pepper flakes and sauté for 5 minutes.

Add the chard and the other ingredients, toss, bring to a simmer and cook over medium heat for 30 minutes more.

Ladle the soup into bowls and serve for lunch.

Nutrition: calories 150, fat 8, fiber 2, carbs 4, protein 9

Hot roasted peppers cream

Preparation time: 10 minutes

Cooking time: 30 minutes

Servings: 4

Ingredients:

1 red chili pepper, minced

4 garlic cloves, minced

2 pounds mixed bell peppers, roasted, peeled and chopped

4 scallions, chopped

1 cup coconut cream

Salt and black pepper to the taste

2 tablespoons olive oil

½ tablespoon basil, chopped

4 cups vegetable stock

¼ cup chives, chopped

Directions:

Heat up a pot with the oil over medium heat, add the garlic and the chili pepper and sauté for 5 minutes.

Add the peppers and the other ingredients, toss, bring to a simmer and cook over medium heat for 25 minutes.

Blend the soup using an immersion blender, divide into bowls and serve.

Nutrition: calories 140, fat 2, fiber 2, carbs 5, protein 8

Eggplant and Peppers Soup

Preparation time: 10 minutes

Cooking time: 40 minutes

Servings: 4

Ingredients:

2 red bell peppers, chopped

3 scallions, chopped

3 garlic cloves, minced

2 tablespoon olive oil

Salt and black pepper to the taste

5 cups vegetable stock

1 bay leaf

½ cup coconut cream

1 pound eggplants, roughly cubed

2 tablespoons basil, chopped

Directions:

Heat up a pot with the oil over medium heat, add the scallions and the garlic and sauté for 5 minutes.

Add the peppers and the eggplants and sauté for 5 minutes more.

Add the remaining ingredients, toss, bring to a simmer, cook for 30 minutes, ladle into bowls and serve for lunch.

Nutrition: calories 180, fat 2, fiber 3, carbs 5, protein 10

Eggplant and Olives Stew

Preparation time: 10 minutes

Cooking time: 30 minutes

Servings: 4

Ingredients:

2 scallions, chopped

2 tablespoons avocado oil

2 garlic cloves, chopped

1 bunch parsley, chopped

Salt and black pepper to the taste

1 teaspoon basil, dried

1 teaspoon cumin, dried

2 eggplants, roughly cubed

1 cup green olives, pitted and sliced

3 tablespoons balsamic vinegar

½ Cup tomato passata

Directions:

Heat up a pot with the oil over medium heat, add the scallions, garlic, basil and cumin and sauté for 5 minutes.

Add the eggplants and the other ingredients, toss, cook over medium heat for 25 minutes more, divide into bowls and serve.

Nutrition: calories 93, fat 1.8, fiber 10.6, carbs 18.6, protein 3.4

Cauliflower and Artichokes Soup

Preparation time: 10 minutes

Cooking time: 25 minutes

Servings: 4

Ingredients:

1 pound cauliflower florets

1 cup canned artichoke hearts, drained and chopped

2 scallions, chopped

2 tablespoons olive oil

2 garlic cloves, minced

6 cups vegetable stock

Salt and black pepper to the taste

2/3 cup coconut cream

2 tablespoons cilantro, chopped

Directions:

Heat up a pot with the oil over medium heat, add the scallions and the garlic and sauté for 5 minutes.

Add the cauliflower and the other ingredients, toss, bring to a simmer and cook over medium heat for 20 minutes more.

Blend the soup using an immersion blender, divide it into bowls and serve.

Nutrition: calories 207, fat 17.2, fiber 6.2, carbs 14.1, protein 4.7

Hot cabbage soup

Preparation time: 10 minutes

Cooking time: 30 minutes

Servings: 4

Ingredients:

3 spring onions, chopped

1 green cabbage head, shredded

2 tablespoons olive oil

1 tablespoon ginger, grated

1 teaspoon cumin, ground

6 cups vegetable stock

Salt and black pepper to the taste

1 teaspoon hot paprika

1 teaspoon chili powder

1 tablespoon cilantro, chopped

Directions:

Heat up a pot with the oil over medium heat, add the spring onions, ginger and the cumin and sauté for 5 minutes.

Add the cabbage and the other ingredients, stir, bring to a simmer and cook over medium heat for 25 minutes more.

Ladle the soup into bowls and serve for lunch.

Nutrition: calories 117, fat 7.5, fiber 5.2, carbs 12.7, protein 2.8

Zucchini muffins

Preparation time: 5 minutes

Cooking time: 30 minutes

Servings: 6

Ingredients:

4 scallions, chopped

1 tablespoon olive oil

2 zucchinis, chopped

1 yellow bell pepper, chopped

Salt and black pepper to the taste

2 tablespoons flaxseed mixed with 3 tablespoons water

1 cup almond flour

1 cup almond milk

1 teaspoon baking powder

2 tablespoons chives, chopped

Directions:

Heat up a pan with the oil over medium heat, add the scallions, zucchini is and the bell pepper and sauté for 5 minutes.

In a bowl, combine the scallions mix with the rest of the ingredients, stir well, divide into a muffin tray and bake at 390 degrees f for 25 minutes.

Divide the muffins between plates and serve them for breakfast.

Nutrition: calories 258, fat 21.8, fiber 4.9, carbs 11.9, protein 6.6

Berry and Dates Oatmeal

Preparation time: 5 minutes

Cooking time: 0 minutes

Servings: 2

Ingredients:

½ cup coconut flesh, unsweetened and shredded

1 cup coconut milk

¼ cup dates, chopped

1 teaspoon vanilla extract

1 tablespoon stevia

1 cup berries, mashed

Directions:

In a bowl, combine the coconut flesh with the coconut milk, the dates and the other ingredients, whisk well, divide into 2 bowls and serve.

Nutrition: calories 572, fat 47.2, fiber 11.5, carbs 38.8, protein 5.8

Tomato oatmeal

Preparation time: 5 minutes

Cooking time: 20 minutes

Servings: 4

Ingredients:

3 cups water

1 cup coconut milk

1 tablespoon avocado oil

1 cup coconut flesh, unsweetened and shredded

¼ cup cherry tomatoes, chopped

A pinch of red pepper flakes

1 teaspoon chili powder

Directions:

Meanwhile, heat up a pan with the oil over medium-high heat, add the tomatoes, chili powder and pepper flakes and sauté for 5 minutes

Add the coconut and sauté for 5 minutes more.

Add the remaining ingredients, toss, bring to a simmer, cook over medium heat fro 10 minutes more, divide into bowls and serve for breakfast.

Nutrition: calories 170, fat 17.8, fiber 1.5, carbs 3.8, protein 1.5

Mushroom muffins

Preparation time: 10 minutes

Cooking time: 30 minutes

Servings: 8

Ingredients:

1 cup cauliflower rice

2 tablespoons flaxseed mixed with 3 tablespoons water

Salt and black pepper to the taste

1 cup cashew cheese, grated

4 scallions, chopped

1 red bell pepper chopped

1 cup white mushrooms, sliced

Cooking spray

Directions:

In a bowl, combine the cauliflower rice with the flaxseed mix, scallions and the other ingredients, and whisk well.

Grease a muffin pan with the cooking spray, divide the mushrooms mix, bake at 350 degrees f for 30 minutes and serve for breakfast.

Nutrition: calories 123, fat 5.6, fiber 1.3, carbs 10.8, protein 7.5

Classic black beans chili

Preparation time: 10 minutes

Cooking time: 3 hours

Servings: 4

Ingredients:

½ cup quinoa

2 and ½ cups veggie stock

14 ounces canned tomatoes, chopped

15 ounces canned black beans, drained

¼ cup green bell pepper, chopped

¼ cup red bell pepper, chopped

A pinch of salt and black pepper

2 garlic cloves, minced

1 carrots, shredded

1 small chili pepper, chopped

2 teaspoons chili powder

1 teaspoon cumin, ground

A pinch of cayenne pepper

½ cup corn

1 teaspoon oregano, dried

For the vegan sour cream:

A drizzle of apple cider vinegar

4 tablespoons water

½ cup cashews, soaked overnight and drained

1 teaspoon lime juice

Directions:

Put the stock in your slow cooker.

Add quinoa, tomatoes, beans, red and green bell pepper, garlic, carrot, salt, pepper, corn, cumin, cayenne, chili powder, chili pepper and oregano, stir, cover and cook on High for 3 hours.

Meanwhile, put the cashews in your blender.

Add water, vinegar and lime juice and pulse really well.

Divide beans chili into bowls, top with vegan sour cream and serve.

Enjoy!

Nutrition: calories 300, fat 4, fiber 4, carbs 10, protein 7

Amazing potato dish

Preparation time: 10 minutes

Cooking time: 3 hours

Servings: 4

Ingredients:

1 and ½ pounds potatoes, peeled and roughly chopped

1 tablespoon olive oil

3 tablespoons water

1 small yellow onion, chopped

½ cup veggie stock cube, crumbled

½ teaspoon coriander, ground

½ teaspoon cumin, ground

½ teaspoon garam masala

½ teaspoon chili powder

Black pepper to the taste

½ pound spinach, roughly torn

Directions:

Put the potatoes in your slow cooker.

Add oil, water, onion, stock cube, coriander, cumin, garam masala, chili powder, black pepper and spinach.

Stir, cover and cook on High for 3 hours.

Divide into bowls and serve.

Enjoy!

Nutrition: calories 270, fat 4, fiber 6, carbs 8, protein 12

Textured Sweet Potatoes and Lentils Delight

Preparation time: 10 minutes

Cooking time: 4 hours and 30 minutes

Servings: 6

Ingredients:

6 cups sweet potatoes, peeled and cubed

2 teaspoons coriander, ground

2 teaspoons chili powder

1 yellow onion, chopped

3 cups veggie stock

4 garlic cloves, minced

A pinch of sea salt and black pepper

10 ounces canned coconut milk

1 cup water

1 and ½ cups red lentils

Directions:

Put sweet potatoes in your slow cooker.

Add coriander, chili powder, onion, stock, garlic, salt and pepper, stir, cover and cook on high for 3 hours.

Add lentils, stir, cover and cook for 1 hour and 30 minutes.

Add water and coconut milk, stir well, divide into bowls and serve right away.

Enjoy!

Nutrition: calories 300, fat 10, fiber 8, carbs 16, protein 10

Incredibly tasty pizza

Preparation time: 1 hour and 10 minutes

Cooking time: 1 hour and 45 minutes

Servings: 3

Ingredients:

For the dough:

½ teaspoon Italian seasoning

1 and ½ cups whole wheat flour

1 and ½ teaspoons instant yeast

1 tablespoon olive oil

A pinch of salt

½ cup warm water

Cooking spray

For the sauce:

¼ cup green olives, pitted and sliced

¼ cup kalamata olives, pitted and sliced

½ cup tomatoes, crushed

1 tablespoon parsley, chopped

1 tablespoon capers, rinsed

¼ teaspoon garlic powder

¼ teaspoon basil, dried

¼ teaspoon oregano, dried

¼ teaspoon palm sugar

¼ teaspoon red pepper flakes

A pinch of salt and black pepper

½ cup cashew mozzarella, shredded

Directions:

In your food processor, mix yeast with italian seasoning, a pinch of salt and flour.

Add oil and the water and blend well until you obtain a dough.

Transfer dough to a floured working surface, knead well, transfer to a greased bowl, cover and leave aside for 1 hour.

Meanwhile, in a bowl, mix green olives with kalamata olives, tomatoes, parsley, capers, garlic powder, oregano, sugar, salt, pepper and pepper flakes and stir well.

Transfer pizza dough to a working surface again and flatten it.

Shape so it will fit your slow cooker.

Grease your slow cooker with cooking spray and add dough.

Press well on the bottom.

Spread the sauce mix all over, cover and cook on high for 1 hour and 15 minutes.

Spread vegan mozzarella all over, cover again and cook on high for 30 minutes more.

Leave your pizza to cool down before slicing and serving it.

Nutrition: calories 340, fat 5, fiber 7, carbs 13, protein 15

Rich beans soup

Preparation time: 10 minutes

Cooking time: 7 hours

Servings: 4

Ingredients:

1 pound navy beans

1 yellow onion, chopped

4 garlic cloves, crushed

2 quarts veggie stock

A pinch of sea salt

Black pepper to the taste

2 potatoes, peeled and cubed

2 teaspoons dill, dried

1 cup sun-dried tomatoes, chopped

1 pound carrots, sliced

4 tablespoons parsley, minced

Directions:

Put the stock in your slow cooker.

Add beans, onion, garlic, potatoes, tomatoes, carrots, dill, salt and pepper, stir, cover and cook on low for 7 hours.

Stir your soup, add parsley, divide into bowls and serve.

Enjoy!

Nutrition: calories 250, fat 4, fiber 3, carbs 9, protein 10

Delicious baked beans

Preparation time: 10 minutes

Cooking time: 12 hours

Servings: 8

Ingredients:

1 pound navy beans, soaked overnight and drained

1 cup maple syrup

1 cup bourbon

1 cup vegan bbq sauce

1 cup palm sugar

¼ cup ketchup

1 cup water

¼ cup mustard

¼ cup blackstrap molasses

¼ cup apple cider vinegar

¼ cup olive oil

2 tablespoons coconut aminos

Directions:

Put the beans in your slow cooker.

Add maple syrup, bourbon, bbq sauce, sugar, ketchup, water, mustard, molasses, vinegar, oil and coconut aminos.

Stir everything, cover and cook on Low for 12 hours.

Divide into bowls and serve.

Enjoy!

Nutrition: calories 430, fat 7, fiber 8, carbs 15, protein 19

Indian lentils

Preparation time: 10 minutes

Cooking time: 3 hours

Servings: 4

Ingredients:

1 yellow bell pepper, chopped

1 sweet potato, chopped

2 and ½ cups lentils, already cooked

4 garlic cloves, minced

1 yellow onion, chopped

2 teaspoons cumin, ground

15 ounces canned tomato sauce

½ teaspoon ginger, ground

A pinch of cayenne pepper

1 tablespoons coriander, ground

1 teaspoon turmeric, ground

2 teaspoons paprika

2/3 cup veggie stock

1 teaspoon garam masala

A pinch of sea salt

Black pepper to the taste

Juice of 1 lemon

Directions:

Put the stock in your slow cooker.

Add potato, lentils, onion, garlic, cumin, bell pepper, tomato sauce, salt, pepper, ginger, coriander, turmeric, paprika, cayenne, garam masala and lemon juice.

Stir, cover and cook on high for 3 hours.

Stir your lentils mix again, divide into bowls and serve. Enjoy!

Nutrition: calories 300, fat 6, fiber 5, carbs 9, protein 12

Delicious butternut squash soup

Preparation time: 10 minutes

Cooking time: 6 hours

Servings: 8

Ingredients:

1 apple, cored, peeled and chopped

½ pound carrots, chopped

1 pound butternut squash, peeled and cubed

1 yellow onion, chopped

A pinch of sea salt

Black pepper to the taste

1 bay leaf

3 cups veggie stock

14 ounces canned coconut milk

¼ teaspoon sage, dried

Directions:

Put the stock in your slow cooker.

Add apple squash, carrots, onion, salt, pepper and bay leaf.

Stir, cover and cook on low for 6 hours.

Transfer to your blender, add coconut milk and sage and pulse really well.

Ladle into bowls and serve right away.

Enjoy!

Nutrition: calories 200, fat 3, fiber 6, carbs 8, protein 10

Amazing mushroom stew

Preparation time: 10 minutes

Cooking time: 8 hours

Servings: 4

Ingredients:

2 garlic cloves, minced

1 celery stalk, chopped

1 yellow onion, chopped

1 and ½ cups firm tofu, pressed and cubed

1 cup water

10 ounces mushrooms, chopped

1 pound mixed peas, corn and carrots

2 and ½ cups veggie stock

1 teaspoon thyme, dried

2 tablespoons coconut flour

A pinch of sea salt

Black pepper to the taste

Directions:

Put the water and stock in your slow cooker.

Add garlic, onion, celery, mushrooms, mixed veggies, tofu, thyme, salt, pepper and flour.

Stir everything, cover and cook on low for 8 hours.

Divide into bowls and serve hot.

Enjoy!

Nutrition: calories 230, fat 4, fiber 6, carbs 10, protein 7

Simple tofu dish

Preparation time: 10 minutes

Cooking time: 3 hours

Servings: 6

Ingredients:

1 big tofu package, cubed

1 tablespoon sesame oil

¼ cup pineapple, cubed

1 tablespoon olive oil

2 garlic cloves, minced

1 tablespoons brown rice vinegar

2 teaspoon ginger, grated

¼ cup soy sauce

5 big zucchinis, cubed

¼ cup sesame seeds

Directions:

In your food processor, mix sesame oil with pineapple, olive oil, garlic, ginger, soy sauce and vinegar and whisk well.

Add this to your slow cooker and mix with tofu cubes.

Cover and cook on High for 2 hours and 45 minutes.

Add sesame seeds and zucchinis, stir gently, cover and cook on High for 15 minutes.

Divide between plates and serve.

Enjoy!

Nutrition: calories 200, fat 3, fiber 4, carbs 9, protein 10

Special jambalaya

Preparation time: 10 minutes

Cooking time: 6 hours

Servings: 4

Ingredients:

6 ounces soy chorizo, chopped

1 and ½ cups celery ribs, chopped

1 cup okra

1 green bell pepper, chopped

16 ounces canned tomatoes and green chilies, chopped

2 garlic cloves, minced

½ teaspoon paprika

1 and ½ cups veggie stock

A pinch of cayenne pepper

Black pepper to the taste

A pinch of salt

3 cups already cooked wild rice for serving

Directions:

Heat up a pan over medium high heat, add soy chorizo, stir, brown for a few minutes and transfer to your slow cooker.

Also, add celery, bell pepper, okra, tomatoes and chilies, garlic, paprika, salt, pepper and cayenne to your slow cooker.

Stir everything, add veggie stock, cover the slow cooker and cook on low for 6 hours.

Divide rice on plates, top each serving with your vegan jambalaya and serve hot.

Enjoy!

Nutrition: calories 150, fat 3, fiber 7, carbs 15, protein 9

Delicious chard soup

Preparation time: 10 minutes

Cooking time: 8 hours

Servings: 6

Ingredients:

1 yellow onion, chopped

1 tablespoon olive oil

1 celery stalk, chopped

2 garlic cloves, minced

1 carrot, chopped

1 bunch Swiss chard, torn

1 cup brown lentils, dried

5 potatoes, peeled and cubed

1 tablespoon soy sauce

Black pepper to the taste

A pinch of sea salt

6 cups veggie stock

Directions:

Heat up a big pan with the oil over medium high heat, add onion, celery, garlic, carrot and Swiss chard, stir, cook for a few minutes and transfer to your slow cooker.

Also, add lentils, potatoes, soy sauce, salt, pepper and stock to the slow cooker, stir, cover and cook on Low for 8 hours.

Divide into bowls and serve hot.

Enjoy!

Nutrition: calories 200, fat 4, fiber 5, carbs 9, protein 12

Chinese Tofu and Veggies

Preparation time: 10 minutes

Cooking time: 4 hours

Servings: 4

Ingredients:

14 ounces extra firm tofu, pressed and cut into medium triangles

Cooking spray

2 teaspoons ginger, grated

1 yellow onion, chopped

3 garlic cloves, minced

8 ounces tomato sauce

¼ cup hoisin sauce

¼ teaspoon coconut aminos

2 tablespoons rice wine vinegar

1 tablespoon soy sauce

1 tablespoon spicy mustard

¼ teaspoon red pepper, crushed

2 teaspoons molasses

2 tablespoons water

A pinch of black pepper

3 broccoli stalks

1 green bell pepper, cut into squares

2 zucchinis, cubed

Directions:

Heat up a pan over medium high heat, add tofu pieces, brown them for a few minutes and transfer to your slow cooker.

Heat up the pan again over medium high heat, add ginger, onion, garlic and tomato sauce, stir, sauté for a few minutes and transfer to your slow cooker as well.

Add hoisin sauce, aminos, vinegar, soy sauce, mustard, red pepper, molasses, water and black pepper, stir gently, cover and cook on high for 3 hours.

Add zucchinis, bell pepper and broccoli, cover and cook on high for 1 more hour.

Divide between plates and serve right away.

Enjoy!

Nutrition: calories 300, fat 4, fiber 8, carbs 14, protein 13

Wonderful corn chowder

Preparation time: 10 minutes

Cooking time: 8 hours and 30 minutes

Servings: 6

Ingredients:

2 cups yellow onion, chopped

2 tablespoons olive oil

1 red bell pepper, chopped

1 pound gold potatoes, cubed

1 teaspoon cumin, ground

4 cups corn kernels

4 cups veggie stock

1 cup almond milk

A pinch of salt

A pinch of cayenne pepper

½ teaspoon smoked paprika

Chopped scallions for serving

Directions:

Heat up a pan with the oil over medium heat, add onion, stir and sauté for 5 minutes and then transfer to your slow cooker.

Add bell pepper, 1 cup corn, potatoes, paprika, cumin, salt and cayenne, stir, cover and cook on low for 8 hours.

Blend this using an immersion blender and then mix with almond milk and the rest of the corn.

Stir chowder, cover and cook on low for 30 minutes more.

Ladle into bowls and serve with chopped scallions on top.

Enjoy!

Nutrition: calories 200, fat 4, fiber 7, carbs 13, protein 16

Black eyed peas stew

Preparation time: 10 minutes

Cooking time: 4 hours

Servings: 8

Ingredients:

3 celery stalks, chopped

2 carrots, sliced

1 yellow onion, chopped

1 sweet potato, cubed

1 green bell pepper, chopped

3 cups black-eyed peas, soaked for 8 hours and drained

1 cup tomato puree

4 cups veggie stock

A pinch of salt

Black pepper to the taste

1 chipotle chile, minced

1 teaspoon ancho chili powder

1 teaspoons sage, dried and crumbled

2 teaspoons cumin, ground

Chopped coriander for serving

Directions:

Put celery in your slow cooker.

Add carrots, onion, potato, bell pepper, black-eyed peas, tomato puree, salt, pepper, chili powder, sage, chili, cumin and stock.

Stir, cover and cook on High for 4 hours.

Stir stew again, divide into bowls and serve with chopped coriander on top.

Enjoy!

Nutrition: calories 200, fat 4, fiber 7, carbs 9, protein 16

White bean cassoulet

Preparation time: 10 minutes

Cooking time: 6 hours

Servings: 4

Ingredients:

2 celery stalks, chopped

3 leeks, sliced

4 garlic cloves, minced

2 carrots, chopped

2 cups veggie stock

15 ounces canned tomatoes, chopped

1 bay leaf

1 tablespoon Italian seasoning

30 ounces canned white beans, drained

For the breadcrumbs:

Zest from 1 lemon, grated

1 garlic clove, minced

2 tablespoons olive oil

1 cup vegan bread crumbs

¼ cup parsley, chopped

Directions:

Heat up a pan with a splash of the veggie stock over medium heat, add celery and leeks, stir and cook for 2 minutes.

Add carrots and garlic, stir and cook for 1 minute more.

Add this to your slow cooker and mix with stock, tomatoes, bay leaf, italian seasoning and beans.

Stir, cover and cook on low for 6 hours.

Meanwhile, heat up a pan with the oil over medium high heat, add bread crumbs, lemon zest, 1 garlic clove and parsley, stir and toast for a couple of minutes.

Divide your white beans mix into bowls, sprinkle bread crumbs mix on top and serve.

Enjoy!

Nutrition: calories 223, fat 3, fiber 7, carbs 10, protein 7

Light jackfruit dish

Preparation time: 10 minutes

Cooking time: 6 hours

Servings: 4

Ingredients:

40 ounces green jackfruit in brine, drained

½ cup agave nectar

½ cup gluten free tamari sauce

¼ cup soy sauce

1 cup white wine

2 tablespoons ginger, grated

8 garlic cloves, minced

1 pear, cored and chopped

1 yellow onion, chopped

½ cup water

4 tablespoons sesame oil

Directions:

Put jackfruit in your slow cooker.

Add agave nectar, tamari sauce, soy sauce, wine, ginger, garlic, pear, onion, water and oil.

Stir well, cover and cook on low for 6 hours.

Divide jackfruit mix into bowls and serve.

Enjoy!

Nutrition: calories 160, fat 4, fiber 1, carbs 10, protein 3

Veggie curry

Preparation time: 10 minutes

Cooking time: 4 hours

Servings: 4

Ingredients:

1 tablespoon ginger, grated

14 ounces canned coconut milk

Cooking spray

16 ounces firm tofu, pressed and cubed

1 cup veggie stock

¼ cup green curry paste

½ teaspoon turmeric

1 tablespoon coconut sugar

1 yellow onion, chopped

1 and ½ cup red bell pepper, chopped

A pinch of salt

¾ cup peas

1 eggplant, chopped

Directions:

Put the coconut milk in your slow cooker.

Add ginger, stock, curry paste, turmeric, sugar, onion, bell pepper, salt, peas and eggplant pieces, stir, cover and cook on high for 4 hours.

Meanwhile, spray a pan with cooking spray and heat up over medium high heat.

Add tofu pieces and brown them for a few minutes on each side.

Divide tofu into bowls, add slowly cooked curry mix on top and serve.

Enjoy!

Nutrition: calories 200, fat 4, fiber 6, carbs 10, protein 9

Chapter 3. Dinner

Noodle Bowl with Creamy Curry Sauce

Servings: 4

Preparation time: 10 min

Cooking time: 2 min

Ingredients:

Kanten noodles – ½ oz

Carrots (julienned) – 2

Cauliflower head (chopped roughly) – ½

Red bell pepper (diced) – 1

Fresh cilantro (chopped) – handful

Mixed greens - 2 handfuls

Sauce:

Tahini – ¼ cup

Apple cider vinegar – 2 tablespoon

Water – ¼ cup

Avocado oil – 2 tablespoon

Curry powder – 2 teaspoon

Ground coriander – 1 ½ teaspoons

Ground turmeric – 1 teaspoon

Ground cumin – 1 teaspoon

Sea salt – 1 teaspoon

Ground black pepper – ½ teaspoon

Ground ginger – ¼ teaspoon

Directions:

Place all the sauce ingredients in a blender and blend until smooth.

For the noodles, place the noodle sheets in a bowl and pour warm water over it. Strain after 5 minutes and place in a large bowl.

Toss together all the ingredients and top with the sauce.

Nutrition: 192 cal, 15.4 g total fat (2.1 g sat. Fat), 7.3 g net carbs, 10.4 g fiber, 4.3 g protein.

Coconut cauliflower rice

Servings: 6

Preparation time: 5 min

Cooking time: 10 min

Ingredients:

Cauliflower (chopped into pieces) – ½

Coconut cream (full-fat) – 1 cup

Shredded coconut (unsweetened) – ¼ cup

Cilantro – 1 teaspoon

Salt to taste

Directions:

Rice the cauliflower using a food processor.

Transfer into a pan over medium flame and mix in the rest of the ingredients.

Cook until softened, stirring occasionally.

Nutrition: 84 cal, 6.9 g total fat, 4.5 g carbs, 1.4g fiber, 2 g protein.

Kelp Noodles with Peanut Butter Sauce

Servings: 4

Preparation time: 10 min

Ingredients:

Kelp noodles – 1 bag

Sauce:

Peanut butter – ½ cup

White onion – 1

Soy sauce – ¼ cup

Lime juice – of 1 lime

Garlic cloves – 3

Red pepper flakes – 2 teaspoon

Directions:

Place all the sauce ingredients in a blender and blend until smooth.

Soak the kelp noodles in water and then drain.

Add ¼ of the sauce on top and serve.

Nutrition: 231 cal, 16 g total fat, 7 g net carbs, 5g fiber, 7 g protein.

Edamame kelp noodles

Servings: 2

Preparation time: 10 min

Cooking time: 10 min

Ingredients:

Kelp noodles – 1 package

Carrots (julienned) – ¼ cup

Edamame (shelled) – ½ cup

Mushrooms (sliced) – ¼ cup

Frozen spinach – 1 cup

Sauce:

Tamari – 2 tablespoon

Sesame oil – 1 tablespoon

Ground ginger – ½ teaspoon

Garlic powder - ½ teaspoon

Sriracha – ¼ teaspoon

Directions:

Soak the kelp noodles in water and then drain.

Place the sauce ingredients in a saucepan over medium flame and then toss in the veggies.

Once warm, add in the noodles.

Simmer covered for a few minutes, stirring occasionally.

Nutrition: 139 cal, 8.6 g total fat, 4.9 g net carbs, 4.5g fiber, 7.8 g protein.

Eggplant lasagna

Servings: 4

Preparation time: 1 hour

Cooking time: 45 min

Ingredients:

Eggplant (slice into rounds) - 1

Salt – 1 tablespoon

Marinara sauce – 1 cup

Vegan cashew ricotta – 1 cup

Vegan cheese (of choice) – ½ cup

Olive oil

Directions:

Salt the eggplant slices and leave aside for an hour.

Rinse the eggplant and pat dry.

Grease a baking dish with olive oil and layer the eggplant slices on them.

Brush some marinara sauce on the slices and sprinkle ¼ cup vegan cheese over.

Spread another layer of eggplant, the ricotta and again spread marinara sauce.

Layer the last layer of eggplant, spread the remaining sauce and finally sprinkle the remaining cheese.

Bake covered for 30 minutes in an oven preheated to 350 degrees Fahrenheit.

Bake uncovered for another 15 minutes.

Nutrition: 142 cal, 8 g total fat, 9 g net carbs, 5g fiber, 5 g protein.

Zucchini Noodles with Avocado Pesto

Servings: 6

Preparation time: 5 min

Cooking time: 2-3 min

Ingredients:

Spiralized zucchini – 2

Olive oil – 1 tablespoon

Cracked bell pepper – to taste

Sauce:

Ripe avocados – 2

Fresh basil leaves – 1 cup

Garlic cloves – 3

Pine nuts – ¼ cup

Lemon juice – 2 tablespoon

Sea salt – ½ teaspoon

Olive oil – ¼ cup

Directions:

Dry the zucchini using paper towels.

Combine all the sauce ingredients in a food processor except the olive oil and pulse until chopped finely and then with the machine running pour in the olive oil gradually until the sauce emulsifies and smoothens.

Heat olive oil in a wok and cook the zucchini noodles in it for 2 minutes.

Place the zucchini noodles in a bowl, add the pesto and pepper and toss together.

Nutrition: 172 cal, 16.1g total fat (2.1 g sat. Fat) , 7.5 g carbs, 3.6g fiber, 2.9 g protein.

Spinach & cucumber tabbouleh

Servings: 6

Preparation time: 10 min

Cooking time: 5 min

Ingredients:

Cauliflower rice – 3 cups

Extra-virgin coconut oil – 2 tablespoon

Salt – 1 teaspoon

Cucumber (peeled, diced) – 1

Cherry tomatoes (chopped) – 1 cup

Spring onions (chopped) – 2

Spinach (chopped) – 3 cups

Parsley (chopped) – 1 cup

Mint (chopped) – ½ cup

Lemon juice – ½ cup

Garlic clove (minced) - 1

Extra-virgin olive oil – ½ cup

Ground black pepper – ¼ teaspoon

Directions:

Heat the coconut oil in a pan and cook the cauliflower rice in it for 5 minutes with a pinch of salt. Set aside.

Whisk together the olive oil, garlic and lemon juice.

Toss the cooked cauliflower rice with the rest of the ingredients including the garlic sauce.

Nutrition: 245 cal, 23.5 g total fat (5.6 g sat. Fat), 8.4 g carb, 3 g fiber, 2.6 g protein.

Basil Zoodles with Olives

Servings: 6

Preparation time: 10 min

Cooking time: 10 min

Ingredients:

Zucchini (spiralized) – 4

Fresh basil – ½ cup

Avocado pesto – ½ cup

Sun-dried tomatoes (drained) – ¼ cup

Kalamata olives (pitted, drained) – 1 cup

Avocados (sliced into strips, seed discarded) – 2

Extra-virgin coconut oil – 2 tablespoon

Salt – ¼ teaspoon

Directions:

Grease a pan with coconut oil and cook the zucchini noodles in it for 2-5 minutes in batches.

Place the zucchini noodles in a bowl and mix in the pesto.

Toss in the rest of the ingredients.

Nutrition: 449 cal, 41.7 g total fat (11.1 g sat. Fat), 19.8 g carb, 11.4 g fiber, 6.3 g protein.

Ginger cauliflower stew

Servings: 6

Preparation time: 10 min

Cooking time: 10 min

Ingredients:

Coconut oil – 2 tablespoons

Onion (chopped finely) – 1

Tomatoes (chopped finely) – 3

Cumin seeds – 1 teaspoon

Cauliflower (separated into florets) – 1 head

Kale (chopped) – 1 cup

Jalapeno (seeded, chopped) – 1

Ginger paste – 2 teaspoons

Cumin powder – 1 tablespoon

Coriander powder – 1 tablespoon

Turmeric powder – 1 teaspoon

Coconut milk (unsweetened, full-fat) – 1 can

Sea salt – 1 teaspoon

Cilantro (chopped) – 2 tablespoon

Directions:

Heat the oil in a pot and add the cumin seeds to it.

Sauté the onions in it for a minute and then mix in the tomatoes.

Cook for a couple of minutes and then stir in the remaining ingredients.

Simmer covered for 15 minutes, stirring in between after every 5 minutes.

Serve the stew.

Nutrition: 204 cal, 24 g total fat, 0 mg chol., 588 mg sodium, 18 g carb, 6 g fiber, 6 g protein.

Veggie soybean chili

Servings: 4

Preparation time: 10 min

Cooking time: 25 min

Ingredients:

Textured vegetable protein – 2.5 oz.

Soy sauce – 1 tablespoon

Vegetable oil – 1 tablespoon

Red bell pepper (diced) – 1

Green bell pepper (diced) – 1

Canned diced tomatoes – 14 oz.

Garlic cloves (minced) – 5

Black soybeans (cooked) – 2 cups

Vegetable broth – ½ cup

Chili powder – ½ teaspoon

Oregano – ½ teaspoon

Smoked paprika powder – ½ teaspoon

Directions:

Place the vegetable protein in a saucepan and submerge it with water.

Mix in the soy sauce and bring to boil, cooking for 5 minutes. Place aside.

Heat oil in a pot and sauté the textured vegetable protein and bell peppers in it for 5 minutes.

Mix in the garlic and stir cook for a minute.

Add the remaining ingredients and bring to boil.

Reduce the flame and cook for 10-15 minutes.

Nutrition: 350 cal, 14 g total fat (2 g sat. Fat), 12 g net carb, 10 g fiber, 28 g protein.

Zoodle primavera

Servings: 2

Preparation time: 5 min

Cooking time: 15 min

Ingredients:

Zucchini (spiralized) - 1

Broccoli florets – 1 cup

Carrot (sliced) – 1

Spinach (chopped) – 1 cup

Snap peas – ½ cup

Shallot (diced) – 1

Olive oil – 2 tablespoon

Garlic cloves (minced) - 2

Italian spices – 2 tablespoons

Lemon zest – 1 teaspoon

Lemon juice – 1 teaspoon

2 oz. Vegan cheese

Salt and pepper to taste

Directions:

Sauté the shallots in a greased pan until translucent.

Mix in the peas, broccoli, spinach, bell pepper and carrots, seasoned with salt and pepper and cook for 5-7 minutes.

Mix in the zucchini and cook for 5 minutes, tossing often.

Add the rest of the ingredients and toss.

Nutrition: 324 cal, 23 g total fat, 20 g carb, 5 g fiber, 13 g protein.

Grilled halloumi salad

Servings: 1 serving

Preparation time: 5 min

Cooking time: 10 min

Ingredients:

Holloumi cheese (sliced) – 3 oz.

Persian cucumber (thinly sliced) – 1

Grape tomatoes (halved) – 5

Baby arugula (washed) – a handful

Walnuts (chopped) – ½ oz.

Salt – to taste

Balsamic vinegar – 1 tablespoon

Olive oil – 1 tablespoon

Directions:

Grill the cheese for 3-5 minutes per side.

Toss together all the ingredients except the cheese.

Top the salad with the grilled cheese slices.

Nutrition: 560 cal, 47 g total fat, 7 g carbs, 21 g protein.

Bell pepper & asparagus salad

Servings: 6

Preparation time: 20 min

Ingredients:

Fresh asparagus (chopped into bite size pieces) – 14 oz

Sweet mini peppers (halved, seeded, sliced thinly) – 17 ½ oz

Red onion (sliced) – 1

Extra-virgin olive oil – ½ cup

Apple cider vinegar – 3 tablespoon

Dijon mustard – 1 tablespoon

Himalayan salt – 1 teaspoon

Cracked bell pepper – 1 teaspoon

Lemon zest – of 1 lemon

Capers (finely chopped) – 2 tablespoon

Rosemary (chopped) – 1 tablespoon

Thyme (chopped) - 1 tablespoon

Walnuts (chopped) – ½ cup

Directions:

Combine all the veggies in a rimmed baking sheet.

Whisk together the rest of the ingredients in a bowl until lightly emulsified.

Pour ¾ of the dressing over the veggies and toss.

Roast for 15 minutes in an oven preheated to 425 degrees Fahrenheit, stirring once or twice.

Then broil the veggies for 5-6 minutes.

Nutrition: 252 cal, 23.4 g total fat (2.8 g sat. Fat), 0 mg chol., 508 mg sodium, 9.2 g carb, 4.1 g fiber, 5 g protein.

Chapter 4. Quick Cooking Recipes

Cauliflower quesadillas

Servings: 4

Preparation time: 20 min

Cooking time: 20 min

Ingredients:

Cauliflower florets (riced in food processor)– 2 lbs.

Eggs - 3

Mozzarella cheese (shredded) – ¾ cup

Sea salt – ½ teaspoon

Mayonnaise – ¼ cup

Jalapenos in water – 1 ½ tablespoon

Paprika – ½ teaspoon

Garlic powder – ¼ teaspoon

Cayenne pepper – 1 pinch

Cheddar cheese (shredded) – 1 cup

Directions:

Whisk together the mayo, paprika, cayenne pepper, garlic powder and jalapenos in a bowl to make the sauce. Refrigerate covered overnight.

Place the cauliflower in a bowl with little water and then microwave it for 8-10 minutes. Using a cheese cloth remove maximum moisture.

Place the cauliflower back into the bowl and mix in the Mozzarella cheese, salt and egg.

Line 2 baking sheets with parchment paper and press the cauliflower mixture on it into 4 circles.

Bake until the bottom is golden and edges are dry for around 8-10 minutes.

Flip and bake for another 6 minutes.

Spread the sauce on the quesadillas and sprinkle the Cheddar cheese over it.

Fold it into half and place on a greased pan over low flame for a couple of minutes and then flip and cook until browned.

Nutrition: 397 cal, 29 g total fat (11 g sat. Fat), 211 mg chol., 789 mg sodium, 14 g carbs, 6 g fiber, 22 g protein.

Pesto avocado & tomato salad

Servings: 2

Preparation time: 5 min

Ingredients:

Tomatoes (sliced) - 3

Avocado (deseeded, peeled, sliced) - 2

Kalamata olives - 6

Mozzarella di bufala – 4.4 oz

Pesto – 2 tablespoon

Extra virgin olive oil - 2 tablespoon

Directions:

Toss together all the ingredients in a bowl.

Enjoy!

Nutrition: 581 cal, 50.7 g total fat (12.2 g sat. Fat), 7.6 g carbs, 9 g fiber, 19.2 g protein.

Asian zucchini salad

Servings: 10

Preparation time: 10 min

Ingredients:

Zucchini (thinly spiralized) – 1

Cabbage (shredded) – 1 lb.

Sunflower seeds (shelled) – 1 cup

Almonds (sliced) – 1 cup

Avocado oil – ¾ cup oil

Stevia drops – 1 teaspoon

White vinegar – 1/3 cup

Directions:

Toss together the zucchini, cabbage, almonds and sunflower seeds in a bowl.

Whisk together the vinegar, oil and stevia in a bowl.

Add the dressing to the salad and toss.

Refrigerate for 2 hours.

Nutrition: 120 cal, 9.3 g total fat (1 g sat. Fat), 0mg chol., 12 mg sodium, 7.3 g carbs, 3.7 g fiber, 4 g protein

Kale Salad with Olives and Chia Croutons

Servings: 4

Preparation time: 15 minutes

Ingredients

For the crouton:

1/2 cup ground chia seed

1/4 cup coconut flour

1 tbsp. Chopped rosemary

1 tsp baking powder

4 eggs

1/2 cup evoo

Salad:

6 cups kale, torn into pieces

3/4 cup pecans, chopped

1/2 cup kalamata olives, pitted

1 batch creamy lemon rosemary dressing (recipe follows)

Directions

Mix the flours, baking powder and rosemary with a pinch of salt. Combine eggs and oil in a separate bowl, whisking until incorporated. Add the dry ingredients to the wet and stir to combine.

Spread the dough onto a sheet tray lined with a silpat. Spread it to 1/2" thick all around, then bake in a 350f oven until golden.

Cut the croutons into cubes, then toss in olive oil and salt and bake for an additional 10-12 minutes. Reserve.

Toss the ingredients for the salad together with the croutons, then dress the salad lightly with the dressing and serve.

Nutrition:

Net carbs: 19.4g, protein: 7g, fat: 18g, calories: 307kcal.

Curried kale salad

Servings: 4

Preparation time: 15 minutes

Ingredients

1 bulb fennel, stem and core cut, sliced

1 red onion, sliced

2 cups sweet potato, peeled and diced

1 tbsp avocado oil

1 tbsp. Curry powder

1 lemon, juiced

1 bunch kale, chopped and steamed

1 pomegranate, seeds removed

1/2 cup fresh coconut meat, diced

1/4 cup cilantro, minced

2 tbsps. Torn mint

2 tbsp evoo

1/8 tsp sea salt

Directions

In a large bowl, mix the fennel, onion, sweet potato, avocado oil, curry powder, and half of the lemon's juice in a bowl. Season with salt and pepper, and toss to combine. Spread the vegetables on a sheet tray and roast in a 400f oven until they are tender, 40-42 minutes.

In a separate bowl, combine the kale, pomegranate, coconut meat, cilantro and mint. Season and reserve.

Make a simple vinaigrette from the other half of the lemon juice, evoo and salt.

Once the roasted vegetables are cooked, cool them and mix them with the kale. Dress the salad with the vinaigrette and serve. Can be served warm or cold.

Nutrition:

Net carbs: 38.8g, protein: 5.7g, fat: 9.8, calories: 249kcal.

Kale Slaw with Green Goddess Dressing

Servings: 4

Preparation time: 10 minutes

Ingredients

5 cups chopped kale

2 cups broccoli florets, chopped

3/4 cup scallions, bias cut

1 carrot, peeled and grated

1/4 cup pumpkin seeds

Sprouts for garnish

For the dressing:

1/2 avocado, pitted

1/2 cup plain almond milk

2 tbsps. Fresh squeezed lemon juice

2 dates

1 tbsp. Apple cider vinegar

1 tbsp evoo

1 tsp dijon mustard

Directions

Mix the kale, broccoli, scallions and carrots in a large bowl. Season and reserve.

Combine the ingredients for the dressing in a blender, then puree to combine. Season well.

Pour the dressing over the greens and toss to combine. Garnish the salad with the seeds and sprouts.

Nutrition:

Net carbs: 22.7g, protein: 7.7g, fat: 19.9g, calories: 301kcal.

Carrot and Feta Salad

Servings: 1

Preparation time: 15 minutes

Ingredients

2 cups carrots, shredded

1/4 cup goat's milk feta, crumbled

2 tbsps. Dill, roughly chopped

2 lemons, juiced

1 tsp evoo

1 clove garlic, minced

Directions

Combine all of the ingredients in a bowl and season, stirring well so that all components are coated in the sauce.

Let stand, covered, for at least 2 hours, if not longer. The longer you wait, the better the flavor will be.

Nutrition:

Net carbs: 19.3g, protein: 8.7g, fat: 13.5g, calories: 247kcal.

Jelly & peanut butter sandwiches

Servings: 4

Preparation time: 5 min

Cooking time: 2 min

Ingredients:

Eggs - 2

Almond flour – 3 tablespoon

Coconut flour – 1 tablespoon

Butter – 1 tablespoon

Baking powder – ½ teaspoon

Peanut butter – 1 tablespoon

Jelly – ½ tablespoon

Directions:

Mix together all the ingredients except the butter and jelly in a mug.

Microwave for 2 minutes on high.

Remove and slice into 4 pieces.

Spread the butter on 2 slices and jelly on the other two.

Cover the butter slice with the jelly slice to make two sandwiches.

Nutrition: 498 cal, 41 g total fat, 459 mg sodium, 14 g carbs, 6 g fiber, 22 g protein.

Cauliflower with Capers

Servings: 2

Preparation time: 10 minutes

Cooking time: 5 minutes

2 cups cauliflower, cut into 1-inch florets

Salt, as required

2 tablespoons coconut oil

1 teaspoon fresh ginger root, sliced thinly

2 fresh thyme sprigs

2 tablespoon capers

In a pan of the water, add the cauliflower and salt and bring to a boil on medium heat.

Cover and cook for about 10-12 minutes.

Drain well and transfer onto a serving platter.

Meanwhile, in a small skillet, melt the coconut oil over medium-low heat.

Add the ginger and thyme sprigs and swirl the pan occasionally for about 2-3 minutes.

Discard the ginger and thyme sprigs.

Pour the oil over cauliflower and top with the capers.

Serve immediately.

Nutrition: Net Carbs: 3.8g; Calories: 152; Total Fat: 14g; Saturated Fat: 11.9g

Protein: 2.4g; Carbs: 7.6g; Fiber: 3.8g; Sugar: 2.5g

Almond Spinach

Servings: 2

Preparation time: 10 minutes

Cooking time: 5 minutes

1 tablespoon olive oil

6 cups fresh spinach

2 garlic cloves, chopped finely

Salt, as required

2 tablespoons almonds, sliced

In a large skillet, heat the oil over medium-high heat and cook the spinach for about 1 minute, stirring continuously.

Add the garlic and salt and cook or about 2-3 minutes or until wilted.

Stir in almond slices and remove from the heat.

Serve hot.

Nutrition: Net Carbs: 2.7g; Calories: 120; Total Fat: 10.3g; Saturated Fat: 1.3g

Protein: 4g; Carbs: 5.5g; Fiber: 2.8g; Sugar: 0.7g

Sweet & Sour Spinach

Servings: 6

Preparation time: 15 minutes

Cooking time: 15 minutes

1 tablespoon olive oil

1 lemon, seeded sliced thinly

1 yellow onion, chopped

2 garlic cloves, minced

2 pounds fresh spinach, chopped

½ cup scallions, chopped

1 teaspoon Erythritol

 Salt and ground black pepper, as required

In a large skillet, heat the oil over medium heat and cook the lemon slices for about 5 minutes.

With a slotted spoon, remove the lemon slices from skillet and set aside.

In the same skillet, add the onion and garlic and sauté for about 5 minutes.

Add the spinach, scallions, Erythritol, salt and black pepper and cook for 3-4 minutes.

Add lemon slices and mix until well combined.

Serve hot.

Nutrition: Net Carbs: 4.4g; Calories: 67; Total Fat: 3g; Saturated Fat: 0.4g

Protein: 4.8g; Carbs: 8.4g; Fiber: 4g; Sugar: 1.7g

Nutty Brussels Sprout

Servings: 2

Preparation time: 10 minutes

Cooking time: 7 minutes

½ pound Brussels sprouts, halved

1 tablespoon olive oil

1 garlic clove, minced

½ teaspoon red pepper flakes, crushed

Salt and ground black pepper, as required

1 tablespoon fresh lemon juice

1 tablespoon pine nuts

In a large skillet, heat the oil over medium heat and sauté the garlic and red pepper flakes for about 40 seconds.

Stir in the Brussels sprouts, salt and black pepper and sauté for about 4-5 minutes.

Stir in lemon juice and sauté for about 1 minute more.

Stir in the pine nuts and remove from the heat.

Serve hot.

Nutrition: Net Carbs: 6.1g; Calories: 143; Total Fat: 10.5g; Saturated Fat: 1.4g

Protein: 4.7g; Carbs: 11g; Fiber: 4.8g; Sugar: 2.8g

Garlicky Mushrooms

Servings: 2

Preparation time: 10 minutes

Cooking time: 8 minutes

½ tablespoon olive oil

½ pound fresh button mushrooms, sliced thinly

1 teaspoon fresh ginger root, minced

1 teaspoon garlic, minced

1 tablespoon red boat fish sauce

Ground black pepper, as required

1 tablespoon scallion (green part), chopped

In a large skillet, heat the oil over high heat and stir fry the mushrooms for about 5-6 minutes.

Add the remaining ingredients except the scallion and stir fry for about 1-2 minutes.

Serve hot with the garnishing pf scallion.

Nutrition: Net Carbs: 3.3g; Calories: 66; Total Fat: 3.9g; Saturated Fat: 0.5g

Protein: 5.7g; Carbs: 4.6g; Fiber: 1.3g; Sugar: 2g

Soy Sauce Green Beans

Servings: 4

Preparation time: 10 minutes

Cooking time: 5 minutes

1 pound fresh green beans, trimmed

Salt, as required

1 tablespoon low-sodium soy sauce

1 tablespoon fresh lime juice

1 tablespoon olive oil

1 tablespoon fresh ginger root, minced

1 tablespoon garlic, minced

¼ teaspoon red pepper flakes

In a pan of the lightly salted boiling water, add the green beans and boil for about 1 minute.

Drain the green beans well and rinse under cold running water.

Place the green beans onto a kitchen towel to dry completely.

In a flat-bottomed skillet, heat the oil over high heat and sauté the ginger and garlic for about 20-30 seconds.

Add the green beans and stir to combine.

Stir in the soy sauce and lime juice and stir fry for about 1-2 minutes.

Remove from the heat and serve.

Nutrition: Net Carbs: 5.3g; Calories: 67; Total Fat: 3.1g; Saturated Fat: 1.9g

Protein: 2.5g; Carbs: 9.3g; Fiber: 4g; Sugar: 1.9g

Green Beans with Tomatoes

Servings: 8

Preparation time: 15 minutes

Cooking time: 40 minutes

¼ teaspoon fresh lemon peel, grated finely

2 teaspoons olive oil

Salt and ground white pepper, as required

4 cups grape tomatoes

1½ pounds fresh green beans, trimmed

Preheat the oven to 350 degrees F.

In a large bowl, mix together lemon peel, oil, salt and white pepper.

Add the cherry tomatoes and toss to coat well.

Transfer the tomato mixture into a roasting pan.

Roast for about 35-40 minutes, stirring once in the middle way.

Meanwhile, in a pan of boiling water, arrange a steamer basket.

Place the green beans in steamer basket and steam, covered for about 7-8 minutes.

Drain the green beans well.

Divide the green beans and tomatoes onto serving plates and serve.

Nutrition: Net Carbs: 5.6g; Calories: 53; Total Fat: 1.5g; Saturated Fat: 0.2g

Protein: 2.3g; Carbs: 9.6g; Fiber: 4g; Sugar: 3.6g

Herbed Asparagus

Servings: 4

Preparation time: 15 minutes

Cooking time: 10 minutes

2 tablespoons olive oil

2 tablespoons fresh lemon juice

1 tablespoon balsamic vinegar

1 teaspoon garlic, minced

1 tablespoon fresh parsley, chopped

1 teaspoon dried oregano

Salt and ground black pepper, as required

1 pound fresh asparagus, ends removed

Preheat the oven to 400 degrees F. Lightly grease a rimmed baking sheet.

In a bowl, add the oil, lemon juice, vinegar, garlic, herbs, salt and black pepper and beat until well combined.

Arrange the asparagus onto the prepared baking sheet in a single layer.

Top with half of the herb mixture and toss to coat.

Roast for about 8-10 minutes.

Remove from the oven and transfer the asparagus onto a platter.

Drizzle with the remaining herb mixture and serve.

Nutrition: Net Carbs: 2.5g; Calories: 88; Total Fat: 7.3g; Saturated Fat: 1.1g

Protein: 2.7g; Carbs: 5.1g; Fiber: 2.6g; Sugar: 2.4g

Zoodles in Tomato Sauce

Servings: 4

Preparation time: 15 minutes

Cooking time: 13 minutes

2 tablespoons olive oil

1 small yellow onion, sliced thinly

2 small garlic clove, minced

¼ teaspoon red pepper flakes, crushed

4 small zucchinis, spiralized with blade C

¼ cup sugar-free tomato sauce

2 tablespoons fresh basil, chopped finely

In a large skillet, heat the oil over medium heat and sauté the onion about 4-5 minutes.

Add the garlic and red pepper flakes and sauté for about 1 minute.

Add the zucchini noodles and cook for about 2 minutes.

Stir in the tomato sauce and cook for about 3-5 minutes or until the desired doneness, stirring occasionally.

Remove from the heat and serve hot with the garnishing of basil.

Nutrition: Net Carbs: 7g; Calories: 101; Total Fat: 7.3g; Saturated Fat: 1g

Protein: 1.8g; Carbs: 9g; Fiber: 0.9g; Sugar: 2.8g

Baked Tofu

Servings: 4

Preparation time: 15 minutes

Cooking time: 30 minutes

1/3 cup low-sodium soy sauce

2 tablespoons balsamic vinegar

½ tablespoon garlic, minced

¼ teaspoon cayenne pepper

1 (16-ounce) package extra-firm tofu, drained, pressed and cubed

½ tablespoon olive oil

1 teaspoon sesame seeds, toasted

1 tablespoon fresh cilantro, chopped

4 cups fresh baby greens

For the tofu in a large bowl, add the soy sauce, vinegar, garlic and cayenne pepper and mix until well combined. Add the tofu cubes and coat with the garlic mixture generously.

Cover the bowl and refrigerate for at least 4 hours.

Preheat the oven to 400 degrees F. Generously, grease a large baking sheet.

Remove the tofu cubes from the bowl and discard the excess marinade.

Arrange the tofu cubes onto the prepared baking sheet in a single layer.

Bake for about 15 minutes per side.

Remove from the oven and set aside for about 5 minutes before serving.

Divide the tofu onto serving plates and garnish with sesame seeds and cilantro.

Serve alongside the greens.

Nutrition: Net Carbs: 3.9g; Calories: 136; Total Fat: 8.8g; Saturated Fat: 0.9g

Protein: 13.1g; Carbs: 4.9g; Fiber: 1g; Sugar: 2.3g

Veggie Burgers

Servings: 6

Preparation time: 20 minutes

Cooking time: 37 minutes

1 tablespoon olive oil

½ of yellow onion, chopped

8 ounces fresh mushrooms, chopped

1 garlic clove, minced

½ teaspoon dried rosemary, crushed

2 cups cauliflower, grated

6 tablespoons almond flour

Salt and ground black pepper, as required

6 cups lettuce, torn

In a skillet, heat the oil over medium heat and sauté onion for about 2 minutes.

Add the mushrooms, garlic and rosemary and sauté for about 3-4 minutes.

Add the cauliflower, salt and black pepper and sauté for about 1 minute.

Remove from heat and transfer mixture into a bowl.

Set aside to cool completely.

Preheat the oven to 400 degrees F. Line a baking sheet with parchment paper.

In the bowl of mushroom mixture, add the almond flour, 2 tablespoons at a time and mix until well combined.

Make 6 equal sized patties from mixture.

Arrange patties onto the prepared baking sheet and bake for about 30 minutes.

Serve hot alongside lettuce.

Nutrition: Net Carbs: 4.7g; Calories: 89; Total Fat: 6.1g; Saturated Fat: 0.6g

Protein: 3.7g; Carbs: 7.3g; Fiber: 2.6g; Sugar: 2.7g

Zucchini Lettice Wraps

Servings: 4

Preparation time: 15 minutes

Cooking time: 13 minutes

1 tablespoon olive oil

1 teaspoon cumin seeds

1 small yellow onion, sliced thinly

4 cups zucchini, grated

½ teaspoon red pepper flakes, crushed

Salt and ground black pepper, as required

8 large lettuce leaves, rinsed and pat dried

2 tablespoons fresh chives, minced finely

In a medium skillet, heat the oil over medium-high heat and sauté the cumin seeds for about 1 minute.

Add the onion and sauté for about 4-5 minutes.

Add the zucchini and cook for about 5-7 minutes or until done completely, stirring occasionally.

Stir in the red pepper flakes, salt and black pepper and remove from the heat.

Arrange the lettuce leaves onto a smooth surface.

Divide the zucchini mixture onto each lettuce leaf evenly.

Top with the chives and serve immediately.

Nutrition: Net Carbs: 4.4g; Calories: 60; Total Fat: 3.9g; Saturated Fat: 0.6g

Protein: 1.8g; Carbs: 6.2g; Fiber: 1.8g; Sugar: 2.9g

Veggies Lettuce Wraps

Servings: 3

Preparation time: 15 minutes

¾ cup fresh kale, tough ribs removed and sliced thinly

½ of avocado, peeled, pitted and chopped

 ¾ cup cucumber, chopped

2 tablespoons scallions, chopped

Salt and ground black pepper, as required

6 large lettuce leaves, rinsed and pat dried

In a large bowl, add the kale, avocado, cucumber, scallion, salt and black pepper and mix well.

Arrange the lettuce leaves onto a smooth surface.

Divide the avocado mixture onto each lettuce leaf evenly.

Serve immediately.

Nutrition: Net Carbs: 3.4g; Calories: 83; Total Fat: 6.6g; Saturated Fat: 1.4g

Protein: 1.4g; Carbs: 6.2g; Fiber: 2.8g; Sugar: 0.8g

Chapter 5. Fancy Recipes

Mexican Lentil Soup

Serving: 6

Nutrition:

233 Cal; 9 g Fat; 1 g Saturated Fat; 32 g Carbohydrates; 10 g Fiber; 13 g Sugars; 9 g Protein;

Preparation time: 10 minutes

Cooking time: 45 minutes

Ingredients:

2 cups green lentils

2 medium carrots, peeled, diced

1 medium red bell pepper, cored, diced

1 avocado, peeled, pitted, and diced

2 celery stalks, diced

1 medium white onion, peeled, diced

2 cups diced tomatoes with their juices

8 ounces diced green chilies

1 tablespoon minced garlic

1/2 teaspoon salt

1 tablespoon cumin

1/4 teaspoon smoked paprika

1 teaspoon oregano

2 tablespoons olive oil

8 cups vegetable broth

Directions:

Take a large pot, place it over medium heat, add oil and when hot, add all the vegetables and cook for 5 minutes until vegetables begin to soften.

Add garlic, stir in oregano, paprika, and cumin, cook for 1 minute until fragrant, then add tomatoes, lentils, and green chilies, season with salt, pour in the broth and bring the mixture to a simmer.

Then cover the pot with lid, and simmer the soup for 30 minutes until lentils have turned tender.

Ladle soup into bowls, top with avocado and cilantro and then serve.

Black Bean and Quinoa Balls with Zucchini Noodles

Serving: 4

Nutrition:

269.2 Cal; 8 g Fat; 1.2 g Saturated Fat; 10 g Carbohydrates; 10.8 g Fiber; 4.4 g Sugars; 13.2 g Protein;

Preparation time: 15 minutes

Cooking time: 40 minutes

Ingredients:

4 zucchinis

For the Balls:

12 ounces of cooked black beans

½ cup quinoa

¼ cup oat flour

¼ cup sesame seeds

1 ½ tablespoon chopped basil

1 teaspoon garlic powder

2 tablespoons nutritional yeast

½ teaspoon ground black pepper

1 teaspoon salt

½ tablespoon Sriracha

2 tablespoons tomato paste

For the Tomato Sauce:

½ cup basil

½ cup sun-dried tomatoes

1 clove of garlic, peeled

½ cup cherry tomato halves

2 tablespoons nutritional yeast

½ teaspoon ground black pepper

2/3 teaspoon salt

1 teaspoon oregano

2 tablespoons toasted pine nuts

1 tablespoon apple cider vinegar

To Serve:

½ cup cherry tomato halves

½ cup chopped basil

Directions:

Prepare the balls and for this, take a medium pot, place it over medium heat, pour in 1 cup water, add quinoa, and cook for 15 minutes until done.

Meanwhile, take a large bowl, add black beans in it, mash them with a fork, add remaining ingredients for the balls in it and stir until combined.

Switch on the oven, then set it to 400 degrees F and let it preheat.

When quinoa has cooked, drain it, let cool for 5 minutes, then add to the bowl containing black beans mixture and mix well until mix until incorporated and the dough comes together.

Shape the dough into balls, about twenty-two, arrange them on a baking sheet lined with baking paper and then bake for 35 to 40 minutes until golden brown on all sides and crispy.

Prepare the tomato sauce, and for this, place all of its ingredients in a food processor and pulse for 2 minutes until smooth.

Prepare the zucchini noodles and for this, spiralized them and placed noodles in a large bowl.

Add tomato sauce to the zucchini noodles, toss until mixed, and then distribute among serving plates.

Top the noodles evenly with baked balls and then serve.

Lentil Meatballs

Serving: 6

Nutrition:

176 Cal; 6 g Fat; 0 g Saturated Fat; 20 g Carbohydrates; 2 g Fiber; 0 g Sugars; 8 g Protein;

Preparation time: 10 minutes

Cooking time: 30 minutes

Ingredients:

For the Balls:

1 ½ cups green lentil, cooked

1 shallot, minced

1 tablespoon minced garlic

1 tablespoon flaxseed meal

¼ cup parsley, chopped

1 tablespoon whole-wheat breadcrumbs

1/3 teaspoon ground black pepper

1 ½ tablespoon Italian seasoning

1 teaspoon salt

2 tablespoons and 1 teaspoon olive oil, divided

1 tablespoon tomato paste

1/3 cup grated vegan parmesan cheese

2 ½ tablespoons water

To Serve:

16 ounces cooked spaghetti, whole-wheat

Directions:

Take a small bowl, place the flaxseed meal in it, then stir in water and let the mixture stand for 5 minutes until thickened.

Switch on the oven, then set it to 375 degrees F and let it preheat.

Meanwhile, take a large skillet pan, place it over medium heat, add 1 tablespoon oil and when hot, add shallot and garlic and cook for 3 minutes until golden brown.

Transfer shallot mixture into a food processor, add remaining ingredients including flaxseed mixture and pulse for 2 minutes until combined.

Shape the mixture into small balls, arrange them onto a baking sheet lined with parchment paper, spray oil over the balls and then bake them for 15 minutes until cooked and golden brown.

Serve meatballs over the cooked spaghetti.

Black Bean Burgers

Serving: 4

Nutrition:

508 Cal; 8 g Fat; 1 g Saturated Fat; 87 g Carbohydrates; 17 g Fiber; 7 g Sugars; 22 g Protein;

Preparation time: 35 minutes

Cooking time: 6 minutes

Ingredients:

½ cup oats, quick-cook

12 ounces cooked black beans

1 medium white onion, peeled, minced

2 medium carrots, shredded

1 tablespoon minced garlic

1/3 teaspoon ground black pepper

½ teaspoon salt

¼ teaspoon cayenne pepper

½ teaspoon red chili powder

½ teaspoon coriander

1 teaspoon cumin

1 tablespoon soy sauce

2 tablespoons olive oil

To Serve:

4 whole-wheat buns, halved, toasted

Directions:

Take a medium skillet pan, place it over medium heat, add 1 tablespoon oil and when hot, add onion and garlic, season with salt and black pepper and cook for 5 minutes.

Then add carrots, stir in cayenne pepper, cumin, red chili powder, and coriander and continue cooking for 5 minutes until tender.

Take a medium bowl, place black beans in it, mash them with a form, add cooked vegetable mixture along with remaining ingredients and stir until incorporated and well mixed.

Shape the mixture into four patties, and then freeze them for 30 minutes.

When ready to cook, take a frying pan, add remaining oil in it, and when hot, add patties and then cook for 3 minutes per side until golden brown and cooked.

Sandwich patties between burger buns and then serve.

Smoked Tofu with Puy Lentils

Serving: 4

Nutrition:

300 Cal; 6 g Fat; 1 g Saturated Fat; 38 g Carbohydrates; 12 g Fiber; 8 g Sugars; 24 g Protein;

Preparation time: 5 minutes

Cooking time: 10 minutes

Ingredients:

18 ounces cooked puy lentils

8 ounces smoked tofu, diced

1 large zucchini, diced

2 red onions, peeled, chopped

2 medium roasted red pepper, sliced

½ cup frozen pea

1 teaspoon smoked paprika

3 tablespoons balsamic vinegar

2 tablespoons olive oil

Directions:

Take a large skillet pan, place it over medium heat, add oil and when hot, add tofu pieces and zucchini, sprinkle with paprika and cook for 4 minutes until zucchini has softened.

Meanwhile, take a medium bowl, place lentils in it, add onion and red pepper, and toss until mixed.

Stir vinegar into the tofu, cook for 2 minutes until reduced slightly, then spoon tofu-zucchini mixture over lentils and toss until just mixed.

Serve straight away.

Black Bean Chili

Serving: 4

Nutrition:

339 Cal; 10 g Fat; 1 g Saturated Fat; 50 g Carbohydrates; 8 g Fiber; 20 g Sugars; 17 g Protein;

Preparation time: 10 minutes

Cooking time: 30 minutes

Ingredients:

28 ounces cooked black beans

2 large white onions, peeled, chopped

28 ounces chopped tomatoes

1 tablespoon minced garlic

2/3 teaspoon ground black pepper

1 1/2 teaspoon salt

3 tablespoons paprika

2 tablespoons brown sugar

3 tablespoons ground cumin

2 tablespoons olive oil

3 tablespoons apple cider vinegar

For Topping:

1 medium avocado, pitted, diced

½ cup chopped green onions

1 radish, peeled, sliced

4 tablespoons vegan sour cream

2 cups of boiled rice

Directions:

Take a large pot, place it over medium heat, add oil and when hot, add onion and garlic and cook for 5 minutes or until softened.

Stir in paprika and cumin, cook for 2 minutes, add tomatoes, black pepper, salt, and sugar, stir until mixed, and continue cooking for 10 minutes.

Add black beans, stir until mixed and cook for 10 minutes.

Distribute rice among bowls, top with prepared chili, then top evenly with avocado, green onions, radish, and sour cream and serve.

Lentil Lasagna

Serving: 4

Nutrition:

378 Cal; 6 g Fat; 1 g Saturated Fat; 63 g Carbohydrates; 10 g Fiber; 11 g Sugars; 19 g Protein;

Preparation time: 15 minutes

Cooking time: 1 hour and 15 minutes

Ingredients:

2 medium cauliflower, cut into floret

28 ounces cooked lentils

1 celery stick, chopped

1 medium white onion, peeled, chopped

1 carrot, peeled, chopped

1 teaspoon minced garlic

1 teaspoon salt

½ teaspoon ground black pepper

1 teaspoon chopped oregano

¼ teaspoon nutmeg

1 tablespoon cornflour

1 tablespoon olive oil

14 ounces chopped tomato

1 teaspoon mushroom ketchup

2 tablespoons soya milk, unsweetened

1 cup vegetable broth

9 lasagna sheets, egg-free

Directions:

Take a large skillet pan, place it over medium heat, add oil and when hot, add onion, carrot, and celery and cook for 10 minutes until softened.

Add garlic, continue cooking for 2 minutes, add lentils, sprinkle with cornflour, and stir until combined.

Add tomatoes, black pepper, salt, oregano, and ketchup, pour in the broth, stir until mixed and simmer for 15 minutes.

Meanwhile, take a medium pot half full with water, place it over medium heat, bring it to a boil, add cauliflower florets and cook for 10 minutes until tender. Drain the florets, transfer them into a food processor, add nutmeg, pour in milk and pulse for 2 minutes until smooth.

Switch on the oven, then set it to 350 degrees F and let it preheat.

Meanwhile, assemble the lasagna and for this, take an 8 by 12 inches baking dish, spread one-third of the lentil mixture in its bottom, cover lentil with some lasagna layers and then cover with one-third of the cauliflower puree.

Create more layers in the same manner with remaining lentil, lasagna, and cauliflower puree, then cover the baking dish with foil and bake for 45 minutes.

After 45 minutes, uncover the baking dish and continue baking the lasagna for 10 minutes until the top has golden brown.

Cut the lasagna into pieces and then serve.

Ramen

Serving: 4

Nutrition:

340 Cal; 14.2 g Fat; 5.1 g Saturated Fat; 41.6 g Carbohydrates; 3.6 g Fiber; 3.1 g Sugars; 9.3 g Protein;

Preparation time: 10 minutes

Cooking time: 1 hour and 5 minutes

Ingredients:

For the Ramen:

1 tablespoon shiitake mushrooms, dehydrated

3-inch piece of ginger, peeled, diced

2 ½ tablespoon minced garlic

1 medium white onion, peeled, chopped

1 tablespoon white miso paste

2 tablespoons soy sauce

1 tablespoon grapeseed oil

1 teaspoon sesame oil

6 cups vegetable stock

16 ounces ramen noodles, cooked

For the Topping:

8 ounces miso-glazed bok choy

1/2 cup chopped green onion

10 ounces tofu, extra-firm, cubed, seared

Directions:

Take a large pot, place it over medium-high heat, add grapeseed oil and when hot, add onion, ginger, and garlic, and then cook for 8 minutes until onions have golden brown.

Stir in 1 cup vegetable stock to remove browned bits from the bottom of the pot, pour in remaining stock, add mushrooms, stir in soy sauce and bring to a simmer, then switch heat to the low level, and simmer the mixture for 1 hour.

Then stir in miso paste and sesame oil, remove the pot from heat, strain the broth and reserve the mushrooms.

Distribute ramen noodles evenly among bowls, pour in the broth, then top with bok choy, green onion, tofu, and mushrooms and then serve.

BBQ Teriyaki Tofu

Serving: 4

Nutrition:

201 Cal; 8 g Fat; 1 g Saturated Fat; 18 g Carbohydrates; 4 g Fiber; 15 g Sugars; 12 g Protein;

Preparation time: 10 minutes

Cooking time: 15 minutes

Ingredients:

For the Marinade:

1/8 teaspoon ground ginger

2 tablespoons brown sugar

2 tablespoons mirin

4 tablespoons soy sauce

1 teaspoon sesame oil

For the Tofu:

2 zucchini, sliced horizontally

12 ounces of tofu, firm, pressed, sliced

7 ounces broccoli florets

2 teaspoons sesame oil

½ tablespoon rapeseed oil

2 teaspoons black sesame seeds

2 teaspoons white sesame seeds

Directions:

Prepare the marinade and for this, take a small bowl, place all of its ingredients in it and then whisk until combined.

Brush the marinade on the slices of tofu until coated, place them in a shallow dish, pour remaining marinade over them and let them marinate for a minimum of 1 hour.

Take a griddle pan, place it over medium heat, whisk together rapeseed oil and sesame oil, brush oil on all sides of zucchini slices and broccoli, then place them on the griddle pan and cook for 7 to 10 minutes until tender.

Place tofu slices on the griddle pan, and then cook for 5 minutes per side until evenly brown and crisp.

Transfer vegetable and tofu slices to a serving dish, drizzle with remaining marinade, sprinkle with sesame seeds and then serve.

Vegetarian Casserole

Serving: 4

Nutrition:

216 Cal; 5.1 g Fat; 0.7 g Saturated Fat; 31 g Carbohydrates; 9.8 g Fiber; 16.1 g Sugars; 12.3 g Protein;

Preparation time: 10 minutes

Cooking time: 40 minutes

Ingredients:

8.8 ounces cooked lentils

2 zucchini, sliced

1 medium red bell pepper, chopped

2 medium sticks of celery, sliced

1 medium white onion, peeled, chopped

1 medium yellow bell pepper, chopped

28 ounces tomatoes

3 medium carrots, sliced

1 tablespoon minced garlic

1 teaspoon smoked paprika

½ teaspoon ground cumin

1 tablespoon dried thyme

2 sprigs of thyme

1 tablespoon olive oil

2 cups cooked white rice

Directions:

Take a large skillet pan, place it over medium heat, add oil and when hot, add onion and cook for 5 minutes until softened.

Add garlic, carrot, celery and bell pepper, stir in paprika, cumin, and thyme and then cook for 5 minutes.

Add tomatoes, zucchini and thyme sprigs, pour in vegetable stock, stir until mixed, and then cook for 20 minutes until done.

Then remove and discard thyme sprigs, add lentils and simmer for 5 minutes until hot.

Distribute rice among bowl, top with lentils and vegetables, and then serve.

Seitan Soup

Serving: 4

Nutrition:

211 Cal; 5 g Fat; 1 g Saturated Fat; 6 g Carbohydrates;

2 g Fiber; 1 g Sugars; 35 g Protein;

Preparation time: 15 minutes

Cooking time: 20 minutes

Ingredients:

8 ounces of tofu, firm, pressed

6 ounces of wheat gluten

1 teaspoon onion powder

3 tablespoons pea protein powder

2 teaspoons garlic powder

1 teaspoon salt

½ teaspoon ground white pepper

2 teaspoons marmite

6 ½ cups vegetable stock

2 teaspoons miso paste

¾ cup soy milk, unsweetened

Directions:

Place tofu in a food processor, add tofu in it, add onion powder, garlic powder, salt, white pepper, miso, marmite, milk, and pulse for 2 minutes until smooth.

Tip the tofu mixture in a bowl, add protein powder, wheat gluten, and stir until incorporated and the dough comes together.

Transfer the dough to a working space, knead it for 10 minutes and set aside until required.

Take a large pot, place it over medium heat, pour in the stock, and bring it to a simmer.

Meanwhile, flatten the dough and then cut it into ½-inch thick chunks.

Add these chunks into the simmering stock, cook for 20 minutes, then ladle into bowls and serve.

Tempeh Tacos

Serving: 6

Nutrition:

217 Cal; 11 g Fat; 2.6 g Saturated Fat; 20 g Carbohydrates; 4 g Fiber; 2.1 g Sugars; 14 g Protein;

Preparation time: 10 minutes

Cooking time: 5 minutes

Ingredients:

1 cup shredded red cabbage

16 ounces of tempeh, crumbled

1 cup chopped pineapple

1/2 bunch of chopped cilantro

2 tablespoons soy sauce

12 ounces BBQ sauce

12 corn tortillas

Directions:

Take a medium skillet pan, place it over medium-high heat, add tortillas in it and cook for 1 minute per side until hot.

Transfer tortillas to a plate, cover them with a kitchen towel and keep them warm until required.

Place tempeh into the skillet pan, crumble it, cook for 2 minutes until warmed, drizzle with soy sauce, toss until mixed, and cook for 2 minutes until thoroughly heated.

Stir in barbecue sauce, stir until mixed and remove the pan from heat.

Assemble tacos and for this, distribute tempeh mixture evenly among them, top with shredded cabbage, cilantro and pineapple and then serve.

Chickpea Pasta Soup

Serving: 6

Nutrition:

187.6 Cal; 1.4 g Fat; 0.2 g Saturated Fat; 40 g Carbohydrates; 5.8 g Fiber; 6.1 g Sugars; 5.6 g Protein;

Preparation time: 5 minutes

Cooking time: 20 minutes

Ingredients:

1 ½ cups cooked chickpeas

1 small white onion, peeled, chopped

1 bunch of kale, destemmed, chopped

2 celery ribs, diced

2 teaspoons minced garlic

2 teaspoons chopped rosemary, divided

1 teaspoon of sea salt

½ teaspoon ground black pepper

2 tablespoons olive oil

1 cup tomato sauce

6 cups vegetable stock

4 ounces whole-wheat linguine

Directions:

Take a large pot, place it over medium heat, add oil and when hot, add onion, garlic, and celery, stir in 1 teaspoon rosemary and cook for 5 minutes until softened.

Add chickpeas, pour in tomato sauce and vegetable stock, stir until mixed, and bring the mixture to a boil.

Add kale leaves, cook for 5 minutes, add linguine pasta, cook it for 7 to 10 minutes until tender and then remove the pot from heat.

Season soup with salt and black pepper, ladle soup into bowls, garnish with remaining rosemary, and then serve.

Pugliese Greens and Beans

Serving: 4

Nutrition:

320 Cal; 15 g Fat; 4 g Saturated Fat; 26 g Carbohydrates; 7 g Fiber; 1 g Sugars; 18 g Protein;

Preparation time: 10 minutes

Cooking time: 20 minutes

Ingredients:

29 ounces cooked chickpeas

4 ounces vegan meat substitute, diced

1 pound kale, chopped

2 tablespoons minced garlic

½ teaspoon ground black pepper

1 teaspoon salt

2 tablespoons olive oil

1/2 cup vegetable broth

4 slices of whole-grain bread, toasted

Directions:

Take a skillet pan, place it over medium heat, add ½ teaspoon oil and when hot, add vegan meat substitute and cook for 3 minutes until golden brown.

Transfer meat substitute to a plate, set aside until required, then add remaining oil into the pan, add red pepper and garlic and cook for 1 minute until fragrant. Add chickpeas, pour in vegetable broth, increase heat to medium-high level and bring it to a simmer.

Add kale, continue simmering for 10 minutes until most of the liquid has evaporated, then add meat substitute in it.

Season with salt and black pepper, remove the pan from heat and then serve with toasted bread slices.

Red Pasta with Lentils

Serving: 4

Nutrition:

778 Cal; 11.3 g Fat; 2.2 g Saturated Fat; 138.6 g Carbohydrates; 31 g Fiber; 20.8 g Sugars; 33.3 g Protein;

Preparation time: 5 minutes

Cooking time: 10 minutes

Ingredients:

1 ½ cups cooked lentils

16 ounces pasta, whole-wheat, cooked

For the Pasta Sauce:

2 tablespoons minced garlic

1/2 cup diced tomatoes

1/2 cup diced carrots

1 teaspoon red chili flakes

½ teaspoon of sea salt

2 tablespoons dried basil

4 tablespoons coconut sugar

2 tablespoons dried oregano

4 tablespoons tomato paste

2 tablespoons olive oil

30-ounce tomato sauce

2 tablespoons grated vegan parmesan cheese

Directions:

Take a large skillet pan, place it over medium heat, add oil, and when hot, add garlic, tomato, and carrots and cook for 3 minutes.

Then remove skillet pan from heat, add salt, red chili flakes, basil, oregano, sugar, tomato paste, tomato sauce, cheese, and stir until mixed.

Switch heat to medium-low level, taste to adjust seasoning, add lentils, stir until combined, and remove the pan from heat.

Distribute pasta among bowls, top with lentil sauce, garnish with some more cheese and basil, and then serve.

Mushroom Pasta

Serving: 4

Nutrition:

249 Cal; 8.4 g Fat; 1.1 g Saturated Fat; 34 g Carbohydrates; 5.8 g Fiber; 8.8 g Sugars; 12.3 g Protein;

Preparation time: 10 minutes

Cooking time: 20 minutes

Ingredients:

8 ounces Shiitake mushrooms, destemmed, diced

16 ounces white mushrooms, diced

1 teaspoon minced garlic

1/8 teaspoon ground black pepper

1/2 teaspoon salt

½ teaspoon red pepper flakes

1 teaspoon dried oregano

½ cup chopped parsley

6 ounces tomato paste

2 tablespoons olive oil

1 cup red wine

1 cup of vegetable broth

2 tablespoons grated parmesan cheese

8 ounces of red lentil spaghetti, cooked

Directions:

Take a large skillet pan, place it over medium-high heat, add oil and when hot, add garlic and cook for 1 minute fragrant.

Stir in tomato paste, cook for 2 minutes until it starts to caramelize, stir in wine and cook for another 2 minutes.

Add all the mushrooms, stir in black pepper, salt, red pepper flakes, and oregano, switch heat to medium-high level and cook for 10 minutes until mushrooms have cooked.

Pour in broth, bring it to a boil and then remove the pan from heat.

Distribute pasta among plates, top with the mushrooms, sprinkle with cheese and then serve.

Jamaican Lentil and Cannellini Beans Curry

Serving: 4

Nutrition:

313 Cal; 7 g Fat; 5 g Saturated Fat; 47.5 g Carbohydrates; 17 g Fiber; 2 g Sugars; 16 g Protein;

Preparation time: 10 minutes

Cooking time: 20 minutes

Ingredients:

1 ¼ cup cooked chickpeas

1/2 cup red lentils

1 medium white onion, peeled, sliced

1 cup spinach

½ of green Chile, chopped

1 ½ tablespoon minced garlic

3/4 teaspoon salt

2 teaspoons Jamaican Curry powder

1/2 teaspoons turmeric powder

½ teaspoon cayenne pepper

1 lemon, cut into wedges

1 teaspoon olive oil

1 cup of coconut milk, unsweetened

1 1/4 cup water

2 tablespoons chopped cilantro

2 cups cooked rice

Directions:

Take a medium skillet pan, place it over medium heat, add oil and when hot, add onion, green chili, and garlic, cook for 4 minutes, or until softened.

Add salt, and all the spices, stir until mixed, cook for 2 minutes until fragrant, add lentils, pour in water and milk, and bring it to a boil.

Add lentils, stir until mixed, cook for 10 minutes until lentils have thoroughly cooked, add spinach and continue cooking for 3 minutes until tender.
Distribute rice among the plate, top with the lentil curry and serve with lemon wedges.

Chapter 6. After Workout

Farro Protein Bowl

Serving: 2

Nutrition:

360 Cal; 11 g Fat; 3 g Saturated Fat; 54.7 g Carbohydrates; 9.5 g Fiber; 11.3 g Sugars; 10.6 g Protein;

Preparation time: 10 minutes

Cooking time: 25 minutes

Ingredients:

1/2 cup farro, uncooked

4 ounces smoky tempeh strips

1 cup diced sweet potatoes

2 cups mixed greens

12 ounces cooked chickpeas

1 cup diced carrots

1/3 teaspoon ground black pepper

2/3 teaspoon salt

2 tablespoons roasted almonds

2 teaspoons olive oil, divided

1/4 cup hummus

1 1/4 cups water

4 lemon, cut into wedges

Directions:

Switch on the oven, then set it to 375 degrees F and let it preheat.

Meanwhile, take a medium bowl, place sweet potato and carrots in it, drizzle with 1 teaspoon oil, season with half of each salt and black pepper, toss until mixed and then spread the vegetables on a third of a large baking sheet.

Add chickpeas into the same bowl, drizzle with the remaining oil, season with remaining salt and black pepper, toss until well coated and spread the chickpeas on second-third of the baking sheet.

Arrange tempeh strips on the remaining space of the baking sheet and then roast it, chickpeas and vegetables for 30 minutes, stirring vegetables and flipping tempeh strips halfway.

Meanwhile, cook the farro beans and for this, take a medium pot, place it over medium-high heat, add farro grains in it, stir in a pinch of salt, pour in water and bring to a boil.

Then cover the pot with a lid, switch heat to medium-low level and cook for 25 minutes until grains have turned soft.

When farro has cooked, distribute evenly between two bowls, top with roasted tempeh, chickpeas, sweet potatoes, and hummus, sprinkle with almonds, and then serve with lemon wedges.

Serve straight away.

Teriyaki Tofu with Quinoa

Serving: 4

Nutrition:

411 Cal; 11 g Fat; 1 g Saturated Fat; 58 g Carbohydrates; 8 g Fiber; 12 g Sugars; 19 g Protein;

Preparation time: 10 minutes

Cooking time: 20 minutes

Ingredients:

For the Tofu:

2 cups diced asparagus

14 ounces tofu, firm, pressed, ½-inch cubed

2 tablespoons chopped green onions

2 teaspoons red chili paste

1 tablespoon soy sauce

2 teaspoons olive oil

For the Sauce:

2 tablespoons minced garlic

2 teaspoons corn starch

1/2 tablespoon grated ginger

1/4 cup coconut sugar

1 tablespoon sesame oil

3 tablespoons soy sauce

1 ½ tablespoon rice vinegar

1/2 cup water

For Serving:

4 cups cooked quinoa

Directions:

Prepare the tofu and for this, take a medium skillet pan, place it over medium-high heat, add 1 teaspoon of olive oil and when hot, add tofu pieces and then cook for 5 minutes until golden brown on all sides.

Then transfer tofu pieces to a bowl, drizzle with soy sauce, toss until coated, and set aside until required.

Prepare the sauce and for this, take a small bowl, place all of its ingredients in it and whisk until combined.

Return skillet pan over medium-high heat, add remaining oil and when hot, add asparagus and then cook for 5 to 7 minutes until tender-crisp.

Return tofu pieces into the pan, drizzle with prepared sauce, toss until well combined, then switch heat to medium level and cook for 3 to 4 minutes until the sauce has thickened.

Add green onions and red chili paste, stir until mixed, and then remove the pan from heat.

Remove pan from heat, then distribute quinoa among serving bowls, top with tofu and vegetables, and serve.

Buddha Bowl

Serving: 2

Nutrition:

503 Cal; 23 g Fat; 5 g Saturated Fat; 61 g Carbohydrates; 13 g Fiber; 9 g Sugars; 18 g Protein;

Preparation time: 10 minutes

Cooking time: 20 minutes

Ingredients:

For the Bowl:

8 ounces tofu, firm, pressed,

1 ½ cups cooked quinoa

1 medium white onion, peeled, sliced

1 cup spinach

1 medium sweet potato, peeled, cubed

¼ cup shredded carrots

1 avocado, pitted, diced

1 cup cooked chickpeas

1 teaspoon minced garlic

1 teaspoon garlic powder

1 teaspoon ground black pepper

1 teaspoon salt

1 teaspoon red chili powder

2 tablespoons olive oil

1 lemon, juiced

For the Marinade:

½ teaspoon salt

1 teaspoon hot sauce

1 teaspoon paprika

2 teaspoons dried thyme

2 tablespoons olive oil

½ teaspoon sesame oil

Directions:

Switch on the oven, then set it to 400 degrees F and let it preheat.

Prepare the bowl and for this, take a small bowl, place all of its ingredients in it and then whisk until combined.

Cut tofu into ½-inch cubes, place them in a container, pour in prepared marinade, toss until well coated, and then marinate tofu pieces for 30 minutes.

Take a large baking sheet, place onion, sweet potato and garlic in it, drizzle with 1 tablespoon oil, season with half of each black pepper and salt, toss until combined, and then bake for 20 minutes until cooked.

Prepare the chickpeas and for this, take a medium bowl, add chickpeas in it, add remaining salt and black pepper, garlic powder and chili powder and stir until combined.

Take a medium skillet pan, place it over medium heat, add remaining oil and when hot, add chickpeas in it and cook for 10 minutes until done.

Transfer chickpeas to a plate, add marinated tofu pieces in it and cook for 10 minutes per side until golden brown, set aside until required.

When vegetables have roasted, take a medium-large bowl, add tofu, quinoa, chickpeas, spinach, sweet potatoes, avocado, onion, and carrots, drizzle with lemon juice and toss until just mixed.

Serve straight away.

Chinese Tofu and Broccoli

Serving: 4

Nutrition:

206 Cal; 8 g Fat; 3 g Saturated Fat; 23 g Carbohydrates; 5 g Fiber; 11 g Sugars; 14 g Protein;

Preparation time: 10 minutes

Cooking time: 20 minutes

Ingredients:

3 cups broccoli florets

14 ounces tofu, firm, pressed, ½-inch cubed

1 teaspoon minced garlic

1 teaspoon grated ginger

1 tablespoon cornstarch

2 tablespoons agave syrup

1 tablespoon rice vinegar

1 teaspoon olive oil

¼ cup of soy sauce

1 ½ teaspoons sesame oil, divided

1 tablespoon water

3 tablespoons vegetable broth

1 teaspoon toasted sesame seeds and more for serving

4 tablespoons sliced scallions

2 cups cooked white rice

Directions:

Take a large skillet pan, place it over medium-high heat, add olive oil and 1 teaspoon sesame oil, and when hot, add tofu pieces and cook for 4 minutes per side until golden brown.

When done, transfer the tofu pieces to a plate, add broccoli florets to the pan, pour in the broth, switch heat to medium-low level and cook for 5 minutes until broccoli has steamed, covering the pan.

Then switch heat to medium-high level, stir in ginger, garlic, and remaining sesame oil and cook for 1 minute. Stir together cornstarch and water until smooth, add to the pan along with sesame seeds, vinegar, agave syrup, and soy sauce, stir until mixed and cook for 2 minutes until the sauce has thickened.

Return tofu pieces to the skillet pan, toss until well coated with the sauce and then remove the pan from heat.

Distribute cooked rice among bowls, top with tofu and broccoli, sprinkle with scallion and sesame seeds and then serve.

Peanut Butter Tempeh with Rice

Serving: 4

Nutrition:

608 Cal; 24 g Fat; 8 g Saturated Fat; 56 g Carbohydrates; 5 g Fiber; 12 g Sugars; 43 g Protein;

Preparation time: 3 hours and 10 minutes

Cooking time: 30 minutes

Ingredients:

6.5 ounces brown rice, cooked

22 ounces Tempeh, 1-inch cubed

Olive oil as needed

For the Sauce:

4 teaspoons coconut sugar

2 tablespoons grated ginger

1 tablespoon minced garlic

2 tablespoons red chili sauce

4 tablespoons soy sauce

2 teaspoons rice vinegar

4 tablespoons peanut butter

6 tablespoons water

For the Cabbage:

1 lime, juiced

5 ounces purple cabbage, sliced

3 teaspoons sesame oil

2 teaspoons honey

For Garnish:

4 tablespoons chopped Green onion

Directions:

Prepare the sauce and for this, take a large bowl, place all of its ingredients in it and whisk until combined.

Add tempeh pieces into the peanut butter sauce, toss until well coated, then place the bowl in the refrigerator and let it marinate for a minimum of 3 hours.

When tofu is almost marinated, switch on the oven, then set the temperature to 375 degrees F and let it preheat.

Transfer marinated tempeh pieces to a baking sheet, spray with olive oil and then bake for 30 minutes until nicely browned and cooked, turning halfway.

Meanwhile, prepare the cabbage and for this, take a medium bowl, place all of its ingredients in it and toss until combined, set aside until required.

When tempeh has baked, distribute cabbage, rice and tempeh pieces evenly among bowls, drizzle with the marinade sauce, garnish with green onions and then serve.

Soy Beans and Puy lentil Salad

Serving: 4

Nutrition:

302 Cal; 7 g Fat; 1 g Saturated Fat; 42 g Carbohydrates; 8 g Fiber; 9 g Sugars; 22 g Protein;

Preparation time: 10 minutes

Cooking time: 25 minutes

Ingredients:

For the Salad:

8 ounces of broccoli florets, chopped

1 red chili, deseeded, sliced

8 ounces of Puy lentils, uncooked

5 ounces sugar snap peas

5 ounces frozen soya bean, thawed

4 ¼ cups vegetable stock, hot

For the Dressing:

1-inch piece of ginger, grated

½ teaspoon minced garlic

1 lemon, juiced

1 tablespoon honey

3 tablespoons soy sauce

2 tablespoons sesame oil

Directions:

Take a large pot, place it over medium-high heat, pour in the stock, bring it to a boil, then add lentils and cook for 15 minutes until tender.

Drain the cooked lentils, transfer them to a large bowl and set aside until required.

Drain the pot, fill it half-full with water, bring it to a boil, then add broccoli florets and cook for 1 minute.

Add soya beans and peas, continue cooking for 1 minute, then drain these vegetables, rinse under cold water and transfer them to the bowl containing lentils. Prepare the dressing and for this, take a small bowl, place all of its ingredients in it and whisk until combined.

Pour the dressing over lentil and vegetable mixture, add red chili, and stir until well mixed.

Serve straight away.

Tofu and Greens Stir-Fry with Cashews

Serving: 4

Nutrition:

358 Cal; 23 g Fat; 3 g Saturated Fat; 13 g Carbohydrates; 6 g Fiber; 8 g Sugars; 25 g Protein;

Preparation time: 5 minutes

Cooking time: 8 minutes

Ingredients:

5 ounces soya bean

1 bunch of spring onions, sliced

2 heads of bok choi, quartered

1 head broccoli, cut into florets

10 ounces of marinated tofu pieces

1 red chili, deseeded, sliced

2 teaspoons minced garlic

1 tablespoon soy sauce

1 ½ tablespoon hoisin sauce

1 tablespoon olive oil

1 ½ tablespoon roasted cashew

Directions:

Take a large skillet pan, place it over high heat, add oil and when hot, add broccoli florets and cook for 5 minutes until tender.

Stir in red chili and garlic, continue cooking for 1 minute, add soya beans, spring onions, tofu, and bok choi, and stir-fry for 3 minutes.

Drizzle with soy sauce and hoisin sauce, sprinkle with nuts, cook for 1 minute until hot and then serve.

Spiced Crusted Tofu with Salad

Serving: 2

Nutrition:

528 Cal; 33 g Fat; 5 g Saturated Fat; 24 g Carbohydrates; 12 g Fiber; 13 g Sugars; 27 g Protein;

Preparation time: 10 minutes

Cooking time: 15 minutes

Ingredients:

For the Tofu:

8 ounces of tofu, firmed, pressed, 1-inch cubed

4 ounces sugar snap peas

3 kumquats, sliced

4 radishes, sliced

8 ounces broccoli florets

2 spring onions, chopped

1 tablespoon Japanese spice mix

2 tablespoons sesame seeds

½ tablespoon cornflour

1 tablespoon sesame oil

1 tablespoon olive oil

For the Dressing:

1 small shallot, diced

1 teaspoon grated ginger

1 tablespoon lime juice

1 teaspoon caster sugar

2 tablespoons soy sauce

1 tablespoon grapefruit juice

Directions:

Prepare the dressing and for this, take a small bowl, place all of its ingredients in it and then stir until well combined.

Prepare the tofu and for this, take a small bowl, add cornflour in it, stir in Japanese spice mix and sesame seeds, and then sprinkle this mixture on all sides of tofu pieces until evenly coated.

Take a large pot, fill it half full with water, place it over high heat, bring it to a boil, then switch heat to medium level, add peas and broccoli and boil for 3 minutes until tender-crisp.

While water comes to a boil, take a large skillet pan, place it over medium heat, add oil and when hot, add tofu pieces and cook for 5 minutes until nicely browned. When Vegetables have cooked to the desired level, distribute them evenly between two bowls, top with cooked tofu, and then drizzle with prepared dressing.

Top with spring onions, radishes, and kumquats and then serve.

Sprouts with Green Beans and Nuts

Serving: 4

Nutrition:

280 Cal; 12 g Fat; 2 g Saturated Fat; 28 g Carbohydrates; 12 g Fiber; 28 g Sugars; 10 g Protein;

Preparation time: 5 minutes

Cooking time: 12 minutes

Ingredients:

21 ounces Brussels sprouts, quartered

21 ounces green beans

4 tablespoons toasted pine nuts

1 lemon, juiced, zested

1 tablespoon olive oil

Directions:

Take a large pot, fill it half full with water, place it over high heat, bring it to a boil, then switch heat to medium level, add beans and sprouts, and boil for 3 minutes until tender-crisp and when done, drain the beans and sprouts.

Take a large skillet pan, place it medium heat, add oil and when hot, add nuts and lemon zest and cook for 30 seconds.

Then add sprouts and green beans, stir-fry them for 4 minutes, then season with black pepper and salt and drizzle with lemon juice.

Remove pan from heat and then serve.

Tofu with Noodles

Serving: 2

Nutrition:

972 Cal; 35 g Fat; 2 g Saturated Fat; 113 g Carbohydrates; 6 g Fiber; 12 g Sugars; 50 g Protein;

Preparation time: 25 minutes

Cooking time: 25 minutes

Ingredients:

8 ounces of tofu, firm, pressed, 1-inch cubed

6 ounces dried soba noodles, cooked

½ of a large cucumber

¼ teaspoon salt

2 tablespoons caster sugar

2 tablespoons sesame seeds

4 tablespoons white miso paste

½ cup of rice wine vinegar

2 tablespoons maple syrup

½ cup olive oil

¼ cup of water

2 spring onions, shredded

Directions:

Prepare the noodles, and for this, use a vegetable peeler to cut ribbons from the cucumber and place them in a bowl.

Take a small saucepan, place it over medium heat, add sugar, salt, vinegar, and water, stir until combined, and cook for 5 minutes until the sugar has dissolved.

Pour this mixture over cucumber ribbons, then place the bowl in the refrigerator and leave it to pickle.

Prepare the tofu and for this, take a large skillet pan, add 1 tablespoon oil in it and when hot, add tofu pieces and cook for 7 to 10 minutes until nicely golden brown on all sides.

When done, transfer the tofu pieces to a plate lined with kitchen towels and then set aside until required.

Take a small bowl, add honey and miso paste in it, whisk until combined, and then brush this mixture on tofu pieces until evenly coated.

When cucumber ribbons have pickles, drain them, and then rinse them well under cold water.

Return the skillet pan over medium heat and when hot, add remaining oil, cucumber ribbons, remaining honey-miso mixture and 1 tablespoon of the cucumber pickling liquid and continue cooking for 3 minutes until warm.

When done, divide soba noodles between bowls, then top evenly with tofu and cucumber ribbons, sprinkle with green onions, and then serve.

Black Bean and Seitan Stir-Fry

Serving: 4

Nutrition:

326 Cal; 8 g Fat; 1 g Saturated Fat; 37 g Carbohydrates; 7 g Fiber; 23 g Sugars; 22 g Protein;

Preparation time: 15 minutes

Cooking time: 25 minutes

Ingredients:

For the Sauce:

1 red chili, chopped

12 ounces cooked black beans

1 tablespoon minced garlic

1 teaspoon Chinese five-spice powder

2.5 ounces brown sugar

2 tablespoons rice vinegar

2 tablespoons soy sauce

1 tablespoon peanut butter

¼ cup of water

For the Stir-Fry:

12 ounces marinated seitan pieces

2 spring onions, sliced

10 ounces bok choi, chopped

1 red pepper, sliced

1 tablespoon cornflour

3 tablespoons olive oil

2 cups cooked brown rice

Directions:

Prepare the sauce, and for this, place half of the black beans in a food processor, then add remaining ingredients and pulse for 2 minutes until smooth.

Tip the sauce in a medium saucepan, place it over medium heat, cook for 5 minutes until thickened, and then set aside until required.

Drain the marinated seitan, pat dries the seitan pieces with kitchen towels, then dredge seitan into cornflour and set aside until required.

Take a large skillet pan, place it over high heat, add 1 teaspoon oil and when hot, add seitan pieces and fry them for 5 minutes until edges have turned golden brown.

When done, transfer seitan pieces to a plate and set aside until required.

Add 1 teaspoon oil into the skillet pan, add shallots, cook for 4 minutes until softened, then add red pepper, spring onion, bok choi, and remaining black beans, stir until mixed and cook for 4 minutes.

Return seitan pieces into the pan, pour in the prepared sauce, toss until mixed, and cook for 1 minute until hot. Serve seitan and vegetables over brown rice.

Curried Tofu Wraps

Serving: 4

Nutrition:

994 Cal; 51 g Fat; 25 g Saturated Fat; 73 g Carbohydrates; 11 g Fiber; 17 g Sugars; 54 g Protein;

Preparation time: 10 minutes

Cooking time: 15 minutes

Ingredients:

20 ounces tofu, 1-inch cubed

½ of medium red cabbage, shredded

2 medium white onions, peeled, sliced

1 tablespoon minced garlic

2/3 teaspoon ground black pepper

1 teaspoon salt

2 tablespoons tandoori curry paste

4 tablespoons soy yogurt

2 tablespoons olive oil

3 tablespoons mint sauce

8 whole-wheat chapatti bread

2 limes, quartered

Directions:

Take a large bowl, place shredded cabbage in it, add ¼ teaspoon black pepper, ½ teaspoon salt, curry paste, 1 tablespoon oil, mint sauce, and yogurt, and then toss until well mixed.

Take a large frying pan, place it over medium heat, add remaining oil and when hot, add tofu pieces and cook for 5 minutes until golden brown.

Transfer tofu pieces to a plate, add onion and garlic and cook for 10 minutes until softened.

Then return tofu pieces to the skillet pan, toss until mixed, season with remaining salt and black pepper, and remove pan heat.

Warm the bread, then top with some cabbage, then top with tofu, drizzle with lime juice and serve.

Black Bean Wraps

Serving: 4

Nutrition:

286 Cal; 17.4 g Fat; 2.4 g Saturated Fat; 24.2 g Carbohydrates; 12.4 g Fiber; 5.5 g Sugars; 15.1 g Protein;

Preparation time: 10 minutes

Cooking time: 0 minutes

Ingredients:

For the Salad:

2 cups cooked black beans

1 cob of corn

3 sticks of celery, chopped

2 medium tomatoes, chopped

1 medium carrot, peeled, chopped

1 cup chopped kale

1 medium avocado, pitted, chopped

1 mango, destoned, chopped

½ cup chopped coriander

For the Dressing:

½ of a medium mango

1 teaspoon grated ginger

1/2 teaspoon salt

1 lemon, juiced

3 tablespoons olive oil

1/4 cup water

For the Wraps:

4 large leaves of lettuce

Directions:

Prepare the dressing and for this, place all of its ingredients in a food processor and then pulse for 1 minute until smooth.

Prepare the salad and for this, take a large bowl, place black beans in it along with remaining ingredients and then toss until combined.

Distribute the salad evenly between lettuce leaves, roll them like a wrap, and then serve.

Cauliflower Steak

Serving: 4

Nutrition:

300 Cal; 24 g Fat; 4 g Saturated Fat; 18 g Carbohydrates; 12 g Fiber; 6 g Sugars; 8 g Protein;

Preparation time: 10 minutes

Cooking time: 23 minutes

Ingredients:

2 medium heads of cauliflower, about 2 pounds

1/2 teaspoon paprika

1 teaspoon chopped parsley

1/2 teaspoon ground black pepper

1 teaspoon salt

1/2 teaspoon garlic powder

1/4 cup olive oil

Directions:

Switch on the oven, then set it to 500 degrees F and let it preheat.

Meanwhile, remove the stem from each cauliflower head, cut each cauliflower in half lengthwise, and then use each half into 1 ½-inch thick steak.

Take a rimmed baking sheet, place cauliflower steaks on it, and then drizzle with oil on both sides.

Take a small bowl, add garlic powder in it, stir in black pepper, salt and paprika until mixed and then sprinkle this mixture on both sides of cauliflower steaks.

Cover the baking sheet with foil, then bake for 5 minutes, uncover the baking sheet and continue baking for 18 minutes until toasted, flipping halfway.

When done, garnish cauliflower steaks with parsley and then serve.

Sweet Corn Chili

Serving: 6

Nutrition:

227 Cal; 3 g Fat; 0 g Saturated Fat; 45 g Carbohydrates; 9 g Fiber; 21 g Sugars; 9 g Protein;

Preparation time: 10 minutes

Cooking time: 8 hours

Ingredients:

For the Chili:

28 ounces diced tomatoes with juices

30 ounces cooked kidney beans

2 cups diced white onion

30 ounces cooked chili beans in sauce, undrained

14.5 ounces sliced stewed tomatoes with juices

15 ounces sweet corn

3 teaspoons minced garlic

1/8 teaspoon ground black pepper

2 ½ tablespoons red chili powder

1/2 teaspoon sea salt

1 tablespoon smoked paprika

3.5 tablespoons cumin

1/8 teaspoon cayenne

2 tablespoons olive oil

6 ounces tomato paste

1 cup vegetable broth

For Serving:

½ cup chopped green onion

1 cup tomato salsa

1 lime, quartered

Directions:

Take a medium skillet pan, place it over medium heat, add oil and when hot, add onion and garlic and cook for 10 minutes until onions have softened and nicely golden brown.

Then transfer the onion-garlic mixture into a 4-quarts slow cooker, add remaining ingredients and stir until mixed.

Switch on the slow cooker, shut with lid and then cook for 8 hours at low heat setting until cooked.

When done, distribute the chili into bowls, top with green onion and salsa, and then serve with a lime wedge.

Chickpea Salad Sandwich

Serving: 4

Nutrition:

444 Cal; 15 g Fat; 2 g Saturated Fat; 61 g Carbohydrates; 6 g Fiber; 3 g Sugars; 14 g Protein;

Preparation time: 10 minutes

Cooking time: 0 minutes

Ingredients:

For the Salad:

15-ounce cooked chickpeas, mashed

1 tablespoon diced red onion

1/2 of a medium avocado, pitted, cubed

1 cup cabbage, shredded

1 tablespoon chives, chopped

½ teaspoon minced garlic

1 tablespoon chopped capers

For the Dressing:

1/2 teaspoon dried basil

½ teaspoon ground black pepper

1 teaspoon of sea salt

1 tablespoon mustard

1 teaspoon lemon juice

1 tablespoon olive oil

1/3 cup vegan mayonnaise

For Serving:

4 sandwich rolls, halved

1 cup chopped lettuce

2 tomato, sliced

1 cucumber, sliced

Directions:

Prepare the salad and for this, take a medium bowl, place all of its ingredients in it and then toss until mixed.

Prepare the dressing and for this, take a small bowl, place all of its ingredients in it, stir until well combined, then drizzle dressing over the salad and toss until mixed.

Assemble the sandwich and for this, distribute salad between rolls, top with lettuce, tomato slices, and cucumber slices and then serve.

Chapter 7. Snacks

Roasted pumpkin seeds

Preparation time: 10 minutes

Cooking time: 40 minutes

Servings: 8

Ingredients:

2 tablespoons olive oil

1 teaspoon garlic powder

2 teaspoons smoked paprika

½ teaspoon salt

1 teaspoon dried oregano

2 cups pumpkin seeds

Method:

Preheat your oven to 300 degrees f.

In a bowl, mix the oil, herbs, spices and salt.

Toss the pumpkin seeds in the mixture.

Transfer to a baking pan.

Roast for 40 minutes.

Store in a glass container with lid for up to 3 days.

Nutrition:

Calories: 50

Total fat: 3g

Saturated fat: 0g

Sodium: 27mg

Potassium: 344mg

Carbohydrates: 6g

Fiber: 5g

Sugar: 1g

Protein: 10g

Crackers & tomato salsa

Preparation time: 10 minutes

Cooking time: 0 minute

Servings: 12

Ingredients:

Crackers

1 clove garlic, crushed and minced

Salt and pepper to taste

3 tomatoes, diced

2 tablespoons onion, chopped

2 teaspoons marjoram, chopped

Method:

Arrange crackers on a plate.

In a bowl, mix the remaining ingredients.

Serve crackers with salsa.

Nutrition:

Calories: 5

Total fat: 0.1g

Sodium: 81mg

Potassium: 58mg

Carbohydrates: 1.1g

Fiber: 0.3g

Sugar: 1g

Protein: 0.2g

Cheesy guacamole & veggie dippers

Preparation time: 10 minutes

Cooking time: 0 minutes

Servings: 10

Ingredients:

3 avocados

2 tablespoons freshly squeezed lemon juice

¼ cup chives, chopped

¼ cup goat cheese, crumbled

Salt and pepper to taste

Method:

Mash the avocados using a fork.

Stir in the rest of the ingredients.

Serve with vegetable dippers like carrot sticks and cucumber strips.

Nutrition:

Calories: 106

Total fat: 9.6g

Saturated fat: 1.7g

Cholesterol: 4mg

Sodium: 114mg

Potassium: 301mg

Carbohydrates: 5.6g

Fiber: 4.2g

Sugar: 1g

Protein: 1.8g

Avocado toast

Preparation time: 5 minutes

Cooking time: 0 minutes

Servings: 1

Ingredients:

5 whole-wheat crackers

¼ avocado, thinly sliced

1 tablespoon black olives, sliced

¼ cup tomatoes, chopped

Method:

Top the crackers with avocado, tomatoes and black olives.

Cover with cling wrap and refrigerate for up to 1 day.

Nutrition:

Calories: 211

Total fat: 13.2g

Saturated fat: 1.5g

Sodium: 293mg

Potassium: 424mg

Carbohydrates: 22.9g

Fiber: 6.3g

Sugar: 5g

Protein: 3.8g

Fruit salad

Preparation time: 20 minutes

Cooking time: 0 minute

Servings: 6

Ingredients:

8 oz. cream cheese

1 tablespoon honey

6 oz. Greek yogurt

1 teaspoon orange zest

1 teaspoon lemon zest

1 orange, sliced into sections

3 kiwi, sliced

1 mango, cubed

1 cup fresh blueberries

Method:

Beat the cream cheese using an electric mixer.

Stir in the honey, yogurt, orange zest and lemon zest.

In a glass jar with lid, arrange the fruits in layers.

Top with the cream cheese mixture.

Seal the jar and refrigerate for up to 1 day.

Nutrition:

Calories: 153

Total fat: 19 g

Saturated fat: 3g

Sodium: 211mg

Potassium: 539mg

Carbohydrates: 31g

Fiber: 5g

Sugar: 7g

Protein: 5g

Grilled peaches

Preparation time: 15 minutes

Cooking time: 15 minutes

Servings: 6

Ingredients:

1 cup balsamic vinegar

1 tablespoon honey

⅛ teaspoon ground cinnamon

3 peaches, sliced in half and pitted

2 teaspoons vegetable oil

¼ cup whipped dessert topping

6 gingersnaps, crushed

Method:

Boil vinegar in a pan.

Simmer for 10 minutes.

Remove from the stove.

Stir in the cinnamon and honey.

Coat the peaches with oil.

Grill for 2 minutes per side.

Drizzle the peaches with the vinegar.

Refrigerate for up to 1 day.

Top with the whipped dessert topping and gingersnaps before serving.

Nutrition:

Calories: 135

Total fat: 3.3g

Saturated fat: 1.2g

Sodium: 42mg

Potassium: 251mg

Carbohydrates: 25.2g

Fiber: 1.7g

Sugar: 18g

Protein: 1.5g

Ginger fruit compote

Preparation time: 15 minutes

Cooking time: 6 hours

Servings: 10

Ingredients:

15 oz. pineapple chunks

3 pears, sliced into cubes

¾ cup apricots, sliced into cubes

1 tablespoon tapioca

3 tablespoons orange juice

1 teaspoon ginger, grated

2 cups cherries, pitted and sliced

¼ cup coconut flakes, toasted

Method:

Add all the ingredients except cherries and coconut flakes in the slow cooker.

Cover the pot.

Cook on low for 6 hours.

Add the cherries.

Sprinkle with the coconut flakes.

Nutrition:

Calories: 124

Total fat: 1.2g

Saturated fat: 0.9g

Sodium: 10mg

Potassium: 275mg

Carbohydrates: 29.4g

Fiber: 3.5g

Sugar: 23g

Protein: 1.5g

Summer berries

Preparation time: 20 minutes

Cooking time: 0 minute

Servings: 12

Ingredients:

2 tablespoons orange juice

1 tablespoon honey

1 teaspoon balsamic vinegar

1 tablespoon orange liqueur

2 cups blueberries

2 cups blackberries

1 cup raspberries

1 cup strawberries

Method:

Blend the orange juice, honey, vinegar and liqueur in a
glass jar with lid.

Shake to blend well.

Toss the berries in a food container.

Seal and refrigerate.

Toss the berries in the mixture when ready to serve.

Nutrition:

Calories: 64

Total fat: 1.6g

Saturated fat: 1g

Cholesterol: 3mg

Sodium: 7mg

Potassium: 110mg

Carbohydrates: 12.1g

Fiber: 2.4g

Sugar: 6g

Protein: 0.9g

Roasted grapes & apples

Preparation time: 15 minutes

Cooking time: 30 minutes

Servings: 6

Ingredients:

3 apples, sliced into wedges

2 cups sweet cherries, pitted and sliced

1 cup grapes

2 tablespoons butter

2 teaspoons lemon juice

2 teaspoons honey

½ teaspoon ground cinnamon

¾ cup vanilla ice cream

Method:

Preheat your oven to 375 degrees f.

Toss the fruits in a baking dish.

In a bowl, mix the rest of the ingredients except the ice cream.

Drizzle this mixture over the fruits.

Coat evenly.

Roast for 30 minutes.

Serve with ice cream.

Nutrition:

Calories: 145

Total fat: 3g

Saturated fat: 1g

Cholesterol: 11mg

Sodium: 46mg

Carbohydrates: 30g

Fiber: 4g

Sugar: 23g

Black Bean Lime Dip

Preparation time: 5 minutes

Cooking time: 6 minutes

Servings: 4

Ingredients:

15.5 ounces cooked black beans

1 teaspoon minced garlic

½ of a lime, juiced

1 inch of ginger, grated

1/3 teaspoon salt

1/3 teaspoon ground black pepper

1 tablespoon olive oil

Method:

Take a frying pan, add oil and when hot, add garlic and ginger and cook for 1 minute until fragrant.

Then add beans, splash with some water and fry for 3 minutes until hot.

Season beans with salt and black pepper, drizzle with lime juice, then remove the pan from heat and mash the beans until smooth pasta comes together.

Serve the dip with whole-grain breadsticks or vegetables.

Nutrition:

Calories: 374

Fat: 14 g

Carbs: 46 g

Protein: 15 g

Fiber: 17 g

Beetroot Hummus

Preparation time: 10 minutes

Cooking time: 60 minutes

Servings: 4

Ingredients:

15 ounces cooked chickpeas

3 small beets

1 teaspoon minced garlic

1/2 teaspoon smoked paprika

1 teaspoon of sea salt

1/4 teaspoon red chili flakes

2 tablespoons olive oil

1 lemon, juiced

2 tablespoon tahini

1 tablespoon chopped almonds

1 tablespoon chopped cilantro

Method:

Drizzle oil over beets, season with salt, then wrap beets in a foil and bake for 60 minutes at 425 degrees F until tender.

When done, let beet cool for 10 minutes, then peel and dice them and place them in a food processor.

Add remaining ingredients and pulse for 2 minutes until smooth, tip the hummus in a bowl, drizzle with some more oil, and then serve straight away.

Nutrition:

Calories: 50.1

Fat: 2.5 g

Carbs: 5 g

Protein: 2 g

Fiber: 1 g

Zucchini Hummus

Preparation time: 5 minutes

Cooking time: 0 minute

Servings: 8

Ingredients:

1 cup diced zucchini

1/2 teaspoon sea salt

1 teaspoon minced garlic

2 teaspoons ground cumin

3 tablespoons lemon juice

1/3 cup tahini

Method:

Place all the ingredients in a food processor and pulse for 2 minutes until smooth.

Tip the hummus in a bowl, drizzle with oil and serve.

Nutrition:

Calories: 65

Fat: 5 g

Carbs: 3 g

Protein: 2 g

Fiber: 1 g

Chipotle and Lime Tortilla Chips

Preparation time: 10 minutes

Cooking time: 15 minutes

Servings: 4

Ingredients:

12 ounces whole-wheat tortillas

4 tablespoons chipotle seasoning

1 tablespoon olive oil

4 limes, juiced

Method:

Whisk together oil and lime juice, brush it well on tortillas, then sprinkle with chipotle seasoning and bake for 15 minutes at 350 degrees F until crispy, turning halfway.

When done, let the tortilla cool for 10 minutes, then break it into chips and serve.

Nutrition:

Calories: 150

Fat: 7 g

Carbs: 18 g

Protein: 2 g

Fiber: 2 g

Carrot and Sweet Potato Fritters

Preparation time: 10 minutes

Cooking time: 8 minutes

Servings: 10

Ingredients:

1/3 cup quinoa flour

1½ cups shredded sweet potato

1 cup grated carrot

1/3 teaspoon ground black pepper

2/3 teaspoon salt

2 teaspoons curry powder

2 flax eggs

2 tablespoons coconut oil

Method:

Place all the ingredients in a bowl, except for oil, stir well until combined and then shape the mixture into ten small patties

Take a large pan, place it over medium-high heat, add oil and when it melts, add patties in it and cook for 3 minutes per side until browned.

Serve straight away

Nutrition:

Calories: 70

Fat: 3 g

Carbs: 8 g

Protein: 1 g

Fiber: 1 g

Buffalo Quinoa Bites

Preparation time: 15 minutes

Cooking time: 30 minutes

Servings: 20

Ingredients:

For the Bites:

1 cup cooked quinoa

15 ounces cooked white beans

3 tablespoons chickpea flour

1 medium shallot, peeled, chopped

3 cloves of garlic, peeled

½ teaspoon ground black pepper

1/2 teaspoon salt

1 teaspoon smoked paprika

1/4 cup vegan buffalo sauce

For the Dressing:

1/4 cup chives

2 tablespoons hemp hearts

1 tablespoon nutritional yeast

1 teaspoon garlic powder

1 teaspoon onion powder

1/2 teaspoon salt

½ teaspoon ground black pepper

2 teaspoons dried dill

1 lemon, juiced

1/4 cup tahini

3/4 cup water

Method:

Prepare the bites, and for this, place half of the beans in a food processor, add garlic and shallots, and pulse for 2 minutes until mixture comes together.

Then add all the spices of the bites and buffalo sauce and pulse for 2 minutes until smooth. Add remaining beans along with chickpea flour and quinoa and pulse until just combined.

Tip the mixture in a dish, shape it in the dough, shape it into twenty balls, about the golf-ball size, and bake for 30 minutes at 350 degrees F until crispy and browned, turning halfway.

Meanwhile, prepare the dressing and for this, place all of its ingredients in a food processor and pulse for 2 minutes until smooth.

Serve bites with prepared dressing.

Nutrition:

Calories: 78

Fat: 3 g

Carbs: 9 g

Protein: 4 g

Fiber: 2 g

Tomato and Pesto Toast

Preparation time: 5 minutes

Cooking time: 0 minute

Servings: 4

Ingredients:

1 small tomato, sliced

¼ teaspoon ground black pepper

1 tablespoon vegan pesto

2 tablespoons hummus

1 slice of whole-grain bread, toasted

Hemp seeds as needed for garnishing

Method:

Spread hummus on one side of the toast, top with tomato slices and then drizzle with pesto.

Sprinkle black pepper on the toast along with hemp seeds and then serve straight away.

Nutrition:

Calories: 214

Fat: 7.2 g

Carbs: 32 g

Protein: 6.5 g

Fiber: 3 g

Avocado and Sprout Toast

Preparation time: 5 minutes

Cooking time: 0 minute

Servings: 4

Ingredients:

1/2 of a medium avocado, sliced

1 slice of whole-grain bread, toasted

2 tablespoons sprouts

2 tablespoons hummus

¼ teaspoon lemon zest

½ teaspoon hemp seeds

¼ teaspoon red pepper flakes

Method:

Spread hummus on one side of the toast and then top with avocado slices and sprouts.

Sprinkle with lemon zest, hemp seeds, and red pepper flakes and then serve straight away.

Nutrition:

Calories: 200

Fat: 10.5 g

Carbs: 22 g

Protein: 7 g

Fiber: 7 g

Apple and Honey Toast

Preparation time: 5 minutes

Cooking time: 0 minute

Servings: 4

Ingredients:

½ of a small apple, cored, sliced

1 slice of whole-grain bread, toasted

1 tablespoon honey

2 tablespoons hummus

1/8 teaspoon cinnamon

Method:

Spread hummus on one side of the toast, top with apple slices and then drizzle with honey.

Sprinkle cinnamon on it and then serve straight away.

Nutrition:

Calories: 212

Fat: 7 g

Carbs: 35 g

Protein: 4 g

Fiber: 5.5 g

Chapter 8. Recipes Around the World

Fluffy Deep-Dish Pizza

Servings: 6

Preparation Time: 2 hours and 15 minutes

Ingredients:

12 inch of frozen whole-wheat pizza crust, thawed

1 medium-sized red bell pepper, cored and sliced

5-ounce of spinach leaves, chopped

1 small red onion, peeled and chopped

1 1/2 teaspoons of minced garlic

1/4 teaspoon of salt

1/2 teaspoon of red pepper flakes

1/2 teaspoon of dried thyme

1/4 cup of chopped basil, fresh

14-ounce of pizza sauce

1 cup of shredded vegan mozzarella

Directions:

Place a medium-sized non-stick skillet pan over an average heat, add the oil and let it heat.

Add the onion, garlic and let it cook for 5 minutes or until it gets soft.

Then add the red bell pepper and continue cooking for 4 minutes or until it becomes tender-crisp.

Add the spinach, salt, red pepper, thyme, basil and stir properly.

Cool off for 3 to 5 minutes or until the spinach leaves wilts, and then set it aside until it is called for.

Grease a 4-quarts slow cooker with a non-stick cooking spray and insert the pizza crust in it.

Press the dough into the bottom and spread 1 inch up along the sides.

Spread it with the pizza sauce, cover it with the spinach mixture and then garnish evenly with the cheese.

Sprinkle it with the red pepper flakes, basil leaves and cover it with the lid.

Plug in the slow cooker and let it cook for 1 1/2 hours to 2 hours at the low heat setting or until the crust turns golden brown and the cheese melts completely.

When done, transfer the pizza into the cutting board, let it rest for 10 minutes, then slice to serve.

Nutrition:

Calories:250 Cal, Carbohydrates:25g, Protein:5g, Fats:8g, Fiber:1g.

Incredible Artichoke and Olives Pizza

Servings: 6

Preparation Time: 1 hours and 50 minutes

Ingredients:

12 inch of frozen whole-wheat pizza crust, thawed

1 mushroom, sliced

1/2 cup of sliced char-grilled artichokes

1 small green bell pepper, cored and sliced

2 medium-sized tomatoes, sliced

2 tablespoons of sliced black olives

1/2 teaspoon of garlic powder

1 teaspoon of salt, divided

1/2 teaspoon of dried oregano

2 tablespoons of nutritional yeast

2-ounce cashews

2 teaspoons of lemon juice

3 tablespoon of olive oil, divided

8-ounce of tomato paste

4 fluid ounce of water

Directions:

Place the cashews in a food processor; add the garlic powder, 1/2 teaspoon of salt, yeast, 2 tablespoons of oil, lemon juice, and water.

Mash it until it gets smooth and creamy, but add some water if need be.

Grease a 4 to 6 quarts slow cooker with a non-stick cooking spray and insert the pizza crust into it.

Press the dough in bottom and spread the tomato paste on top of it.

Sprinkle it with garlic powder, oregano and top it with the prepared cashew mixture.

Spray it with the mushrooms, bell peppers, tomato, artichoke slices, olives and then with the remaining olive oil.

Sprinkle it with the oregano, the remaining salt and cover it with the lid.

Plug in the slow cooker and let it cook for 1 to 1 1/2 hours at the low heat setting or until the crust turns golden brown.

When done, transfer the pizza to the cutting board, let it rest for 10 minutes and slice to serve.

Nutrition:

Calories:212 Cal, Carbohydrates:39g, Protein:16g, Fats:5g, Fiber:5g.

Mushroom and Peppers Pizza

Servings: 6

Preparation Time: 2 hours

Ingredients:

12 inch of frozen whole-wheat pizza crust, thawed

1/2 cup of chopped red bell pepper

1/2 cup of chopped green bell pepper

1/2 cup of chopped orange bell pepper

3/4 cup of chopped button mushrooms

1 small red onion, peeled and chopped

1 teaspoon of garlic powder, divided

1 teaspoon of salt, divided

1/2 teaspoon of coconut sugar

1/2 teaspoon of red pepper flakes

1 teaspoon of dried basil, divided

1 1/2 teaspoon of dried oregano, divided

1 tablespoon of olive oil

6-ounce of tomato paste

1/2 cup of vegan Parmesan cheese

Directions:

Place a large non-stick skillet pan over an average heat, add the oil and let it heat.

Add the onion, bell peppers and cook for 10 minutes or until it gets soft and lightly charred. Then add the mushroom, cook it for 3 minutes and set the pan aside until it is needed.

Pour the tomato sauce, sugar, 1/2 teaspoon of the garlic powder, salt, basil, oregano, into a bowl and stir properly.

Grease a 4 to 6 quarts slow cooker with a non-stick cooking spray and insert the pizza crust into it.

Press the dough in bottom and spread the already prepared tomato sauce on top of it. Sprinkle it with the Parmesan cheese and top it with the cooked vegetable mixture.

Cover it with the lid, plug in the slow cooker and let it cook for 1 to 1 1/2 hours at the low heat setting or until the crust turns golden brown.

When done, transfer the pizza to a cutting board, sprinkle it with the remaining oregano, basil, then let it rest for 10 minutes and then slice to serve.

Nutrition:

Calories:188 Cal, Carbohydrates:27g, Protein:5g, Fats:5g, Fiber:3g.

Tangy Barbecue Tofu Pizza

Servings: 6

Preparation Time: 2 hours

Ingredients:

12 inch of frozen whole-wheat pizza crust, thawed

1 cup of tofu pieces

1 small red onion, peeled and sliced

1/4 cup of chopped cilantro

1 1/2 teaspoons of salt

3/4 teaspoon of ground black pepper

1 tablespoon of olive oil

1 cup of barbecue sauce

2 cups of vegan mozzarella

Directions:

Place a large non-stick skillet pan over an average heat, add 1 tablespoon of oil and let it heat.

Add the tofu pieces in a single layer sprinkle it with 1 teaspoon of salt, black pepper and cook for 5 to 7 minutes or until it gets crispy with a golden brown on all sides.

Transfer the tofu pieces into a bowl, add 1/2 cup of the barbecue sauce and toss it properly to coat.

Grease a 4 to 6 quarts slow cooker with a non-stick cooking spray and insert the pizza crust in it.

Press the dough into the bottom and spread the remaining 1/2 cup of the barbecue sauce.

Evenly garnish it with tofu pieces and onion slices.

Sprinkle it with the mozzarella cheese and cover it with the lid.

Plug in the slow cooker and let it cook for 1 to 1 1/2 hours at the low heat setting or until the crust turns golden brown.

When done, transfer the pizza into the cutting board, let it rest for 10 minutes and slice to serve.

Nutrition:

Calories:135 Cal, Carbohydrates:15g, Protein:6g, Fats:5g, Fiber:1g.

Tasty Tomato Garlic Mozzarella Pizza

Servings: 6

Preparation Time: 2 hours and 30 minutes

Ingredients:

12 inch of frozen whole-wheat pizza crust, thawed

3/4 teaspoon of tapioca flour

2 teaspoons of minced garlic

2 teaspoons of agar powder

1 teaspoon of cornstarch

1 teaspoon of salt, divided

1/2 teaspoon of red pepper flakes

1/2 teaspoon of dried basil

1/2 teaspoon of dried parsley

2 tablespoons of olive oil

1/4 teaspoon of lemon juice

3/4 teaspoon of apple cider vinegar

8 fluid ounce of coconut milk, unsweetened

Directions:

Start by preparing the mozzarella.

Place a small saucepan over a medium-low heat, pour in the milk and let it steam until it gets warm thoroughly.

With a whisker, pour in the agar powder and stir properly until it dissolves completely.

Switch the temperature to a low and pour in the salt, lemon juice, vinegar, and whisk them properly.

Mix the tapioca flour and cornstarch with 2 tablespoons of water before adding it to the milk mixture.

Whisk properly and transfer this mixture to a greased bowl.

Place the bowl in a refrigerator for 1 hour or until it is set.

Then grease a- 4 to 6 quarts of the slow cooker with a non-stick cooking spray and insert pizza crust into it.

Press the dough into the bottom and brush the top with olive oil.

Spread the garlic and then cover it with the tomato slices.

Sprinkle it with salt, red pepper flakes, basil, and the oregano.

Cut the mozzarella cheese into coins and place them across the top of the pizza.

Cover it with the lid, plug in the slow cooker, let it cook for 1 to 1 1/2 hours at the low heat setting or until the crust turns golden brown and the cheese melts completely. When done, transfer the pizza to the cutting board, then let it rest for 5 minutes, and slice to serve.

Nutrition:

Calories:113 Cal, Carbohydrates:10g, Protein:7g, Fats:5g, Fiber:1g.

Delicious Chipotle Red Lentil Pizza

Servings: 4

Preparation Time: 1 hours and 45 minutes

Ingredients:

12 inch of frozen whole-wheat pizza crust, thawed

1/4 cup of red lentils, uncooked and rinsed

1/4 cup of chopped carrot

1 cups of chopped tomato

1 medium-sized tomatoes, sliced

2 green onions, sliced

1 chipotle chili pepper in adobo sauce. Chopped

1/2 cup of sliced olives

1/4 cup of chopped red onion

1/2 teaspoon of minced garlic

1/2 teaspoon of salt

1/4 teaspoon of ground black pepper

1/2 teaspoon of cayenne pepper

1/2 teaspoon of dried oregano

1 teaspoon of dried basil, divided

1 tablespoon of tomato paste

1 teaspoon of olive oil

1/2 teaspoon of apple cider vinegar

1 cup of water

1 cup crumbled almond ricotta cheese

Directions:

Place a medium-sized non-stick skillet pan over an average heat, add the oil and let it heat.

Add the onion, garlic and using the sauté button, heat it for 5 minutes or until the onions get soft.

Add the carrots, tomatoes, chipotle chile, oregano, 1/2 teaspoon of basil and stir properly.

Let it cook for 5 minutes before adding the lentils, salt, black pepper, cayenne pepper, vinegar, and water.

Stir properly, cook for 15 to 20 minutes or until the lentils get tender, thereafter, cover the pan partially with a lid.

In the meantime, grease a 4 to 6 quarts slow cooker with a non-stick cooking spray and insert pizza crust into it.

Press the dough into the bottom and spread the lentil mixture.

Spray it with the tomato slices, green onions, and olives.

Spread the cheese over the top and sprinkle it with the remaining 1/2 teaspoon of basil.

Cover it with the lid, plug in the slow cooker and let it cook for 1 hour or until the crust turns golden brown and allow the cheese to melt completely.

When done, transfer the pizza to the cutting board, then let it rest for 5 minutes, before slicing to serve.

Nutrition:

Calories:369 Cal, Carbohydrates:56g, Protein:5g, Fats:15g, Fiber:5g.

Nourishing Whole-Grain Porridge

Servings: 4

Preparation Time: 2 hours and 10 minutes

Ingredients:

3/4 cup of steel-cut oats, rinsed and soaked overnight

3/4 cup of whole barley, rinsed and soaked overnight

1/2 cup of cornmeal

1 teaspoon of salt

3 tablespoons of brown sugar

1 cinnamon stick, about 3 inches long

1 teaspoon of vanilla extract, unsweetened

4 1/2 cups of water

Directions:

Using a 6-quarts slow cooker, place all the ingredients and stir properly.

Cover it with the lid, plug in the slow cooker and let it cook for 2 hours or until grains get soft, while stirring halfway through.

Serve the porridge with fruits.

Nutrition:

Calories:129 Cal, Carbohydrates:22g, Protein:5g, Fats:2g, Fiber:4g.

Pungent Mushroom Barley Risotto

Servings: 4

Preparation Time: 3 hours and 30 minutes

Ingredients:

1 1/2 cups of hulled barley, rinsed and soaked overnight

8 ounces of carrots, peeled and chopped

1 pound of mushrooms, sliced

1 large white onion, peeled and chopped

3/4 teaspoon of salt

1/2 teaspoon of ground black pepper

4 sprigs thyme

1/4 cup of chopped parsley

2/3 cup of grated vegetarian Parmesan cheese

1 tablespoon of apple cider vinegar

2 tablespoons of olive oil

1 1/2 cups of vegetable broth

Directions:

Place a large non-stick skillet pan over a medium-high heat, add the oil and let it heat until it gets hot.

Add the onion along with 1/4 teaspoon of each the salt and black pepper.

Cook it for 5 minutes or until it turns golden brown.

Then add the mushrooms and continue cooking for 2 minutes.

Add the barley, thyme and cook for another 2 minutes.

Transfer this mixture to a 6-quarts slow cooker and add the carrots, 1/4 teaspoon of salt, and the vegetable broth.

Stir properly and cover it with the lid.

Plug in the slow cooker, let it cook for 3 hours at the high heat setting or until the grains absorb all the cooking liquid and the vegetables get soft.

Remove the thyme sprigs, pour in the remaining ingredients except for parsley and stir properly.

Pour in the warm water and stir properly until the risotto reaches your desired state.

Add the seasoning, then garnish it with parsley and serve.

Nutrition:

Calories:321 Cal, Carbohydrates:48g, Protein:12g, Fats:10g, Fiber:11g.

Healthful Lentil and Rice Stew

Servings: 6

Preparation Time: 4 hours and 15 minutes

Ingredients:

1/2 cup of brown rice, rinsed

1 cup of brown lentils, rinsed

1 cup of chopped white onion

3/4 teaspoon of salt

1 teaspoon of ground turmeric

1 tablespoon of ground cumin

1/2 teaspoon of ground cinnamon

1 1/2 tablespoons of olive oil

1 1/2 quarts of water

Directions:

Place a medium-sized non-stick skillet pan over a medium heat, add the oil and let it heat.

Add the onion and using the sauté button, heat it for 5 minutes or until it turns golden brown.

Transfer this mixture to a 6-quarts slow cooker, pour in the remaining ingredients and cover it with the lid.

Plug in the slow cooker and let it cook for 3 to 4 hours at the high heat setting or until the grains get soft.

Garnish it with the cilantro and serve it with lemon wedges.

Nutrition:

Calories:369 Cal, Carbohydrates:56g, Protein:5g, Fats:15g, Fiber:5g.

Remarkable Three-Grain Medley

Servings: 6

Preparation Time: 3 hours and 15 minutes

Ingredients:

1/2 cup of uncooked hulled barley, rinsed and soaked overnight

1/2 cup of uncooked wild rice, rinse and soaked overnight

2/3 cup of uncooked wheat berries, rinsed and soaked overnight

1/2 cup of sliced green onions

1 teaspoon of minced garlic

1/4 cup of chopped parsley

2 teaspoons of shredded lemon peel

1/4 cup of olive oil

28-ounce of vegetable broth

2 ounces of diced cherry pepper

Directions:

Place all the ingredients in a 6-quarts slow cooker and stir properly.

Cover it with the lid, plug in the slow cooker and let it cook for 2 to 3 hours at the high heat setting or until the grains absorbs all the liquid, as a result becoming soft.

Serve right away.

Nutrition:

Calories:200 Cal, Carbohydrates:38g, Protein:5g, Fats:3g, Fiber:3g.

Hearty Millet Stew

Servings: 4

Preparation Time: 4 hours and 30 minutes

Ingredients:

1 cup of millet, uncooked

2 medium-sized potatoes, peeled and chopped

2 medium-sized carrots, peeled and chopped

1 cup of celery, chopped

1/2 pound of mushrooms, chopped

2 medium-sized white onions, peeled and sliced

1 teaspoon of minced garlic

1 teaspoon of salt

1/2 teaspoon of ground black pepper

1/2 teaspoon of dried basil

1/2 teaspoon of dried thyme

2 bay leaves

4 cups of water

Directions:

Place a medium-sized non-stick skillet pan over an average heat, add the millet and let it cook for 5 minutes or until it gets toasted, while stirring frequently.

Transfer the toasted millets to a 6-quarts slow cooker, and reserve the pan.

Add the potatoes, carrots, celery, mushrooms and onion to the pan and let it cook for 5 to 7 minutes or until it is properly toasted.

Transfer the veggies to the slow cooker, pour in the remaining ingredients, stir and cover it with the lid.

Then plug in the slow cooker and let it cook for 4 hours at the high heat setting or until the vegetables and grains are cooked thoroughly.

Serve right away.

Nutrition:

Calories:268 Cal, Carbohydrates:44g, Protein:8g, Fats:6g, Fiber:8g.

Mushroom Steak

Preparation Time: 1 hr. 30 min.

Servings: 8

Nutrition: Calories: 87, Carbohydrates: 6.2 g, Proteins: 3 g, Fats: 6.2 g

Ingredients:

1 tbsp. of the following:

fresh lemon juice

olive oil, extra virgin

2 tbsp. coconut oil

3 thyme sprigs

8 medium Portobello mushrooms

For Sauce:

1 ½ t. of the following:

minced garlic

minced peeled fresh ginger

2 tbsp. of the following:

light brown sugar

mirin

½ c. low-sodium soy sauce

Directions:

For the sauce, combine all the sauce ingredients, along with ¼ cup water into a little pan and simmer to cook. Cook using a medium heat until it reduces to a glaze, approximately 15 to 20 minutes, then remove from the heat.

For the mushrooms, bring the oven to 350 heat setting. Using a skillet, melt coconut oil and olive oil, cooking the mushrooms on each side for about 3 minutes.

Next, arrange the mushrooms in a single layer on a sheet for baking and season with lemon juice, salt, and pepper.

Carefully slide into the oven and roast for 5 minutes.

Let it rest for 2 minutes.

Plate and drizzle the sauce over the mushrooms.

Enjoy.

Spicy Grilled Tofu Steak

Preparation Time: 20 min.

Servings: 4

Nutrition: Calories: 155, Carbohydrates: 7.6 g, Proteins: 9.9 g, Fats: 11.8 g

Ingredients:

1 tbsp. of the following:

chopped scallion

chopped cilantro

soy sauce

hoisin sauce

2 tbsp. oil

¼ t. of the following:

salt

garlic powder

red chili pepper powder

ground Sichuan peppercorn powder

½ t. cumin

1 pound firm tofu

Directions:

Place the tofu on a plate and drain the excess liquid for about 10 minutes.

Slice drained tofu into ¾ thick stakes.

Stir the cumin, Sichuan peppercorn, chili powder, garlic powder, and salt in a mixing bowl until well-incorporated.

In another little bowl, combine soy sauce, hoisin, and 1 teaspoon of oil.

Heat a skillet to medium temperature with oil, then carefully place the tofu in the skillet.

Sprinkle the spices over the tofu, distributing equally across all steaks. Cook for 3-5 minutes, flip, and put spice on the other side. Cook for an additional 3 minutes.

Brush with sauce and plate.

Sprinkle some scallion and cilantro and enjoy.

Piquillo Salsa Verde Steak

Preparation Time: 25 min.

Servings: 8

Nutrition: Calories: 427, Carbohydrates: 67.5 g, Proteins: 14.2 g, Fats: 14.6 g

Ingredients:

4 – ½ inch thick slices of ciabatta

18 oz. firm tofu, drained

5 tbsp. olive oil, extra virgin

Pinch of cayenne

½ t. cumin, ground

1 ½ tbsp. sherry vinegar

1 shallot, diced

8 piquillo peppers (can be from a jar) – drained and cut to ½ inch strips

3 tbsp. of the following:

parsley, finely chopped

capers, drained and chopped

Directions:

Place the tofu on a plate to drain the excess liquid, and then slice into 8 rectangle pieces.

You can either prepare your grill or use a grill pan. If using a grill pan, preheat the grill pan.

Mix 3 tablespoons of olive oil, cayenne, cumin, vinegar, shallot, parsley, capers, and piquillo peppers in a medium bowl to make our salsa verde. Season to preference with salt and pepper.

Using a paper towel, dry the tofu slices.

Brush olive oil on each side, seasoning with salt and pepper lightly.

Place the bread on the grill and toast for about 2 minutes using medium-high heat.

Next, grill the tofu, cooking each side for about 3 minutes or until the tofu is heated through.

Place the toasted bread on the plate then the tofu on top of the bread.

Gently spoon out the salsa verde over the tofu and serve.

Butternut Squash Steak

Preparation Time: 50 min.

Servings: 4

Nutrition: Calories: 300, Carbohydrates: 46 g, Proteins: 5.3 g, Fats: 10.6 g

Ingredients:

2 tbsp. coconut yogurt

½ t. sweet paprika

1 ¼ c. low-sodium vegetable broth

1 sprig thyme

1 finely chopped garlic clove

1 big thinly sliced shallot

1 tbsp. margarine

2 tbsp. olive oil, extra virgin

Salt and pepper to liking

Directions:

Bring the oven to 375 heat setting.

Cut the squash, lengthwise, into 4 steaks.

Carefully core one side of each squash with a paring knife in a crosshatch pattern.

Using a brush, coat with olive oil each side of the steak then season generously with salt and pepper.

In an oven-safe, non-stick skillet, bring 2 tablespoons of olive oil to a warm temperature.

Place the steaks on the skillet with the cored side down and cook at medium temperature until browned, approximately 5 minutes.

Flip and repeat on the other side for about 3 minutes.

Place the skillet into the oven to roast the squash for 7 minutes.

Take out from the oven, placing on a plate and covering with aluminum foil to keep warm.

Using the previously used skillet, add thyme, garlic, and shallot, cooking at medium heat. Stir frequently for about 2 minutes.

Add brandy and cook for an additional minute.

Next, add paprika and whisk the mixture together for 3 minutes.

Add in the yogurt seasoning with salt and pepper.

Plate the steaks and spoon the sauce over the top.

Garnish with parsley and enjoy!

Cauliflower Steak Kicking Corn

Preparation Time: 60 min.

Servings: 6

Nutrition: Calories: 153, Carbohydrates: 15 g, Proteins: 4 g, Fats: 10 g

Ingredients:

2 t. capers, drained

4 scallions, chopped

1 red chili, minced

¼ c. vegetable oil

2 ears of corn, shucked

2 big cauliflower heads

Salt and pepper to taste

Directions:

Heat the oven to 375 degrees.

Boil a pot of water, about 4 cups, using the maximum heat setting available.

Add corn in the saucepan, cooking approximately 3 minutes or until tender.

Drain and allow the corn to cool, then slice the kernels away from the cob.

Warm 2 tablespoons of vegetable oil in a skillet.

Combine the chili pepper with the oil, cooking for approximately 30 seconds.

Next, combine the scallions, sautéing with the chili pepper until soft.

Mix in the corn and capers in the skillet and cook for approximately 1 minute to blend the flavors. Then remove from heat.

Warm 1 tablespoon of vegetable oil in a skillet. Once warm, begin to place cauliflower steaks to the pan, 2 to 3 at a time. Season to your liking with salt and cook over medium heat for 3 minutes or until lightly browned.

Once cooked, slide onto the cookie sheet and repeat step 5 with the remaining cauliflower.

Take the corn mixture and press into the spaces between the florets of the cauliflower.

Bake for 25 minutes.

Serve warm and enjoy!

Pistachio Watermelon Steak

Preparation Time: 10 min.

Servings: 4

Nutrition: Calories: 67, Carbohydrates: 3.8 g, Proteins: 1.6 g, Fats: 5.9 g

Ingredients:

Microgreens

Pistachios chopped

Malden sea salt

1 tbsp. olive oil, extra virgin

1 watermelon

Salt to taste

Directions:

Begin by cutting the ends of the watermelon.

Carefully peel the skin from the watermelon along the white outer edge.

Slice the watermelon into 4 slices, approximately 2 inches thick.

Trim the slices, so they are rectangular in shape approximately 2 x4 inches.

Heat a skillet to medium heat add 1 tablespoon of olive oil.

Add watermelon steaks and cook until the edges begin to caramelize.

Plate and top with pistachios and microgreens.

Sprinkle with Malden salt.

Serve warm and enjoy!

BBQ Ribs

Preparation Time: 45 min.

Servings: 2

Nutrition: Calories: 649, Carbohydrates: 114 g, Proteins: 34.8 g, Fats: 11.1 g

Ingredients:

2 drops liquid smoke

2 tbsp. of the following:

soy sauce

tahini

1 c. of the following:

water

wheat gluten

1 tbsp. of the following:

garlic powder

onion powder

lemon pepper

2 t. chipotle powder

For the Sauce:

2 chipotle peppers in adobo, minced

1 tbsp. of the following:

vegan Worcestershire sauce

lemon juice

horseradish

onion powder

garlic powder

ground pepper

1 t. dry mustard

2 tbsp. sweetener of your choice

5 tbsp. brown sugar

½ c. apple cider vinegar

2 c. ketchup

1 c. water

1 freshly squeezed orange juice

Directions:

Set the oven to 350 heat setting, and prepare the grill charcoal as recommended for this, but gas will work as well.

Combine soy sauce, tahini, water, and liquid smoke in a bowl. Then set this mixture to the side in a mixing bowl.

Next, use a big glass bowl to mix chipotle powder, onion powder, lemon pepper, garlic powder; combine well then whisk in the ingredients from the little bowl.

Add the wheat gluten and mix until it comes to a gooey consistency.

Grease a standard-size loaf pan and transfer the mixture to the loaf pan. Smooth it out so that the rib mixture fits flat in the pan.

Bake for 30 minutes.

While the mixture is baking, make the BBQ sauce. To make the sauce, combine all the sauce ingredients in a pot. Allow the mixture to simmer its way to the boiling point to combine the flavors, and as soon as it boils, decrease the heat to the minimum setting. Let it be for 10 more minutes.

Cautiously take the rib out of the oven and slide onto a plate.

Coat the top rib mixture with the BBQ Sauce and place on the grill.

Coat the other side of the rib mixture with BBQ Sauce and grill for 6 minutes

Flip and grill the other side for an additional 6 minutes.

Serve warm and enjoy!

Spicy Veggie Steaks With veggies

Preparation Time: 45 mins.

Servings: 4

Nutrition: Calories: 458, Carbohydrates: 65.5 g,
Proteins: 39.1 g, Fats: 7.6 g

Ingredients:

1 ¾ c. vital wheat gluten

½ c. vegetable stock

¼ t. liquid smoke

1 tbsp. Dijon mustard

1 t. paprika

½ c. tomato paste

2 tbsp. soy sauce

½ t. oregano

¼ t. of the following:

coriander powder

cumin

1 t. of the following:

onion powder

garlic powder

¼ c. nutritional yeast

¾ c. canned chickpeas

Marinade:

½ t. red pepper flakes

2 cloves garlic, minced

2 tbsp. soy sauce

1 tbsp. lemon juice, freshly squeezed

¼ c. maple syrup

For skewers:

15 skewers, soaked in water for 30 minutes if wooden

¾ t. salt

8 oz. zucchini or yellow summer squash

¼ t. ground black pepper

1 tbsp. olive oil

1 red onion, medium

Directions:

In a food processor, add chickpeas, vegetable stock, liquid smoke, Dijon mustard, pepper, paprika, tomato paste, soy sauce, oregano, coriander, cumin, onion powder, garlic, and natural yeast. Process until the ingredients are well-mixed.

Add the vital wheat gluten to a big mixing bowl, and pour the contents from the food processor into the center. Mix with a spoon until a soft dough is formed.

Knead the dough for approximately 2 minutes; do not over knead.

Once the dough is firm and stretchy, flatten it to create 4 equal-sized steaks.

Individually wrap the steaks in tin foil; be sure not to wrap the steaks too tightly, as they will expand when steaming.

Steam for 20 minutes. To steam, you can use any steamer you like or a basket over boiling water.

While steaming, prepare the marinade. In a bowl, whisk the red pepper, garlic, soy sauce, lemon juice, and syrup. Reserve half of the sauce for brushing during grilling.

Prepare the skewers. Cut the onion and zucchini or yellow squash into 1/2-inch chunks.

In a glass bowl, add the red onion, zucchini, and yellow squash then coat with olive oil, pepper, and salt to taste. Place the vegetables on the skewers.

After the steaks have steamed for 20 minutes, unwrap and place on a cookie sheet. Pour the marinade over the steaks, fully covering them.

Bring your skewers, steaks, and glaze to the grill. Place the skewers on the grill over direct heat. Brush skewers with glaze. Grill for approximately 3 minutes then flip.

Place the steaks directly on the grill, glaze side down, and brush the top with additional glaze. Cook to your desired doneness.

Serve warm and enjoy!

Tofu Seitan

Preparation Time: 1 hr, 40 mins.

Servings: 6

Nutrition: Calories: 159, Carbohydrates: 8 g, Proteins: 26 g, Fats: 2 g

Ingredients:

½ t. salt

1 t. garlic, powdered

2 t. vegetable broth

1 tbsp. onion, powdered

2 tbsp. of the following

nutritional yeast

water

1 ¼ c. tofu

1 ½ c. vital wheat gluten

Directions:

Stir together the ingredients above in a bowl until a dough forms.

Lightly dust the countertop and your hands with wheat gluten. Using the counter service, form a ball out of the dough. Be careful not to knead it because it might make the seitan tough.

Once the ball is formed, cut it into 6 equal pieces.

Using your fingers press each ball into an oval shape, about 4x6 inches.

With a steamer basket placed inside a big pot, add water into the bottom of the pot and bring it to a rolling boil.

Place the seitan into the steamer basket; if they overlap, brush them with oil to prevent them from sticking.

Cover and steam for approximately 12 minutes then flip so that both sides steam evenly.

Once steamed on both sides, remove and allow cooling for a minimum of 1 hour.

The tenders are fully cooked at this point, so you can re-heat them or toss them on the grill with your favorite sauce, or you can eat them cold over leafy greens.

Enjoy!

Stuffed Zucchini

Preparation Time: 30 mins.

Servings: 4

Nutrition: Calories: 159, Carbohydrates: 8 g, Proteins: 26 g, Fats: 2 g

Ingredients:

1 ½ c. black beans, drained

¼ t. chili powder

½ of the following:

sea salt

cumin, ground

1 of the following

clove garlic, minced

red bell pepper, diced

red onion, diced

1 tbsp. olive oil, extra virgin

4 medium zucchini

For the Sauce

¼ t. of the following:

chili powder

turmeric

sea salt

1 tbsp. Nutritional yeast

½ t. apple cider vinegar

¼ c. of the following:

water

raw tahini

4 t. Lemon juice

Directions:

Set the oven to 350 heat setting.

Slice the knobs off the top and bottom of the zucchini, and then slice in half lengthwise.

Scoop the center of the seeds from each zucchini with a spoon, creating a bowl to hold the filling.

On a big cookie sheet, place the zucchini bowls and bake for approximately 20 minutes.

Using a big skillet, combine onion and pepper and sauté for five minutes at medium-high temperature until softened.

Add garlic and sauté for an additional minute.

Turn the skillet down to medium heat and sprinkle in the chili powder, cumin, salt, and black beans and warm. Remove from the stove and cover to maintain warmth.

Prepare the sauce. Using a little bowl, whisk the sauce ingredients until smooth and creamy.

Remove the zucchini from the oven when finished cooking.

Fill each zucchini bowl generously with the bean mixture.

Drizzle the sauce over.

Serve warm and enjoy!

Roasted Butternut Squash With Chimichurri

Preparation Time: 30 mins.

Servings: 2

Nutrition: Calories: 615, Carbohydrates: 71.6 g, Proteins: 12.5 g, Fats: 35.7 g

Ingredients:

1 c. onion, thinly sliced

2 cloves garlic

1 tbsp. coconut oil

1 acorn squash

2 tbsp. olive oil (best if extra virgin)

¼ c. goji berries

1 c. water

2 c. mushrooms, sliced

½ c. quinoa

Chimichurri Sauce

½ t. salt

2 tbsp. lime

½ c. olive oil, extra virgin

¼ t. cayenne pepper

1 shallot

3 cloves garlic

1 tbsp. sherry vinegar

1 c. parsley

Directions:

Bring the broiler to the maximum heat setting.

Stir up the chimichurri sauce by combining the parsley, vinegar, garlic shallot, cayenne pepper, olive oil, lime juice, and ½ cup of olive oil. Blend well; if you want the sauce a little thinner, then add additional extra virgin oil.

Prepare an aluminum-foiled cookie sheet.

Divide the squash in half by carefully cutting widthwise, and remove seeds and pulp from the center.

Cut each half of the squash into moon shape slices; you should get about 4-6 slices.

Place the slices on the aluminum foil sheet and spritz olive oil across the top.

Keep a close eye on the squash; you want nice char marks, nothing more. Once one side is charred to your liking, flip the squash and char the other side.

While broiling, bring a medium-sized saucepan of water to a rolling boil then simmer the quinoa, cooking for 10 minutes or until tender.

Heat a skillet to medium heat, and sauté the onions. Once the onions are caramelizing, add in the mushroom and garlic, cooking on low heat for approximately 5 minutes.

Plate the squash, topping it with quinoa and mushroom.

Sprinkle goji berries across the plate and drizzle chimichurri sauce.

Serve warm and enjoy!

Eggplant Pizza

Preparation Time: 30 mins.

Servings: 8

Nutrition: Calories: 234, Carbohydrates: 27 g, Proteins: 5.4 g, Fats: 12 g

Ingredients:

2 tbsp. olive oil

¼ t. of the following:

pepper

salt

½ t. oregano, dried

1 c. panko

½ tbsp. almond flour

1 tbsp. flaxseed, ground

1/3 c. water

½ eggplant, medium size

2 c. marinara sauce

1 lb. vegan pizza dough

For the cheese:

¼ lb. tofu, extra firm drained

2 tbsp. almond milk, unsweetened

½ c. cashews, soaked for 6 hours, drained

3 tbsp. lemon juice, freshly squeezed

Directions:

Set the oven to 400 heat setting; prepare a cookie sheet with ½ tablespoon of olive oil by brushing to coat.

Whisk together flaxseed, flour, and water in a little bowl.

In a different bowl, combine salt, pepper, oregano, and panko.

Prepare the eggplant by slicing into ¼ inch triangles.

Dip each eggplant triangle into the flaxseed mixture then coat with panko mixture and place on the cookie sheet.

Slide gently into the oven and baking for 15 minutes.

Flip and then bake for an additional 15 minutes or until lightly browned.

Take out of the oven and set to the side.

Get a pizza stone or pizza pan ready for the dough.

Lightly flour the workspace, and with a rolling pin, work the dough to a 14-inch circle then transfer to the pizza stone or pizza pan.

Brush the dough's top with olive oil and slide into the warm oven, cooking until lightly browned or for about twenty minutes.

While the crust is baking, prepare the cheese by placing cashews in the high-speed blender, blending until it reaches a crumbly consistency.

Then add to the blender the lemon juice, almond milk, and tofu; blend until it's a chunky cheese-like consistency. Set to the side.

Once the crust is cooked, assemble the pizza by saucing crust with marinara, adding eggplant slices, and placing the cheese on top.

Serve warm and enjoy!

Green Avocado Carbonara

Preparation Time: 15 mins.

Servings: 1

Nutrition: Calories: 526, Carbohydrates: 24.6 g, Proteins: 5.8 g, Fats: 48.7 g

Ingredients:

Spinach angel hair

Parsley, fresh

2 t. olive oil, extra virgin

2 cloves garlic, diced

½ lemon, zest, and juice

1 avocado, pitted

Salt and pepper to taste

Directions:

Combine using a food processor the parsley, olive oil, garlic, lemon, and avocado and blend until smooth.

Prepare the noodles according to package.

Place noodles in a bowl, and add the sauce on top of noodles.

Add pepper and salt to your liking.

Serve warm and enjoy!

Chapter 9. Low Calories Recipes

Savory Spanish Rice

Servings: 10

Preparation Time: 3 hours and 10 minutes

Ingredients:

1 cup of long grain rice, uncooked

1/2 cup of chopped green bell pepper

14 ounce of diced tomatoes

1/2 cup of chopped white onion

1 teaspoon of minced garlic

1/2 teaspoon of salt

1 teaspoon of red chili powder

1 teaspoon of ground cumin

4-ounce of tomato puree

8 fluid ounce of water

Directions:

Grease a 6-quarts slow cooker with a non-stick cooking spray and add all the ingredients into it.

Stir properly and cover the top.

Plug in the slow cooker; adjust the cooking time to 5 hours and let it cook on the high heat setting or until the rice absorbs all the liquid.

Serve right away.

Nutrition:

Calories:210 Cal, Carbohydrates:11g, Protein:12g, Fats:10g, Fiber:3g.

Exquisite Banana, Apple, and Coconut Curry

Servings: 6

Preparation Time: 6 hours and 10 minutes

Ingredients:

1/2 cup of amaranth seeds

1 apple, cored and sliced

1 banana, sliced

1 1/2 cups of diced tomatoes

3 teaspoons of chopped parsley

1 green pepper, chopped

1 large white onion, peeled and diced

2 teaspoons of minced garlic

1 teaspoon of salt

1 teaspoon of ground cumin

2 1/2 tablespoons of curry powder

2 tablespoons of flour

2 bay leaves

1/2 cup of white wine

8 fluid ounce of coconut milk

1/2 cup of water

Directions:

Using a food processor place the apple, tomatoes, garlic and pulse it until it gets smooth but a little bit chunky.

Add this mixture to a 6-quarts slow cooker and add the remaining ingredients.

Stir until it mixes properly and cover the top.

Plug in the slow cooker; adjust the cooking time to 6 hours and let it cook on the low heat setting or until it is cooked thoroughly.

Add the seasoning and serve right away.

Nutrition:

Calories:370 Cal, Carbohydrates:15g, Protein:5g, Fats:8g, Fiber:8g.

Hearty Vegetarian Lasagna Soup

Servings: 10

Preparation Time: 7 hours and 20 minutes

Ingredients:

12 ounces of lasagna noodles

4 cups of spinach leaves

2 cups of brown mushrooms, sliced

2 medium-sized zucchinis, stemmed and sliced

28 ounce of crushed tomatoes

1 medium-sized white onion, peeled and diced

2 teaspoon of minced garlic

1 tablespoon of dried basil

2 bay leaves

2 teaspoons of salt

1/8 teaspoon of red pepper flakes

2 teaspoons of ground black pepper

2 teaspoons of dried oregano

15-ounce of tomato sauce

6 cups of vegetable broth

Directions:

Grease a 6-quarts slow cooker and place all the ingredients in it except for the lasagna and spinach.

Cover the top, plug in the slow cooker; adjust the cooking time to 7 hours and let it cook on the low heat setting or until it is properly done.

In the meantime, cook the lasagna noodles in the boiling water for 7 to 10 minutes or until it gets soft.

Then drain and set it aside until the slow cooker is done cooking.

When it is done, add the lasagna noodles into the soup along with the spinach and continue cooking for 10 to 15 minutes or until the spinach leaves wilts.

Using a ladle, serving it in a bowl.

Nutrition:

Calories:188 Cal, Carbohydrates:13g, Protein:18g, Fats:9g, Fiber:0g.

Tastiest Barbecued Tofu and Vegetables

Servings: 4

Preparation Time: 4 hours 15 minutes

Ingredients:

14-ounce of extra-firm tofu, pressed and drained

2 medium-sized zucchini, stemmed and diced

1/2 large green bell pepper, cored and cubed

3 stalks of broccoli stalks

8 ounce of sliced water chestnuts

1 small white onion, peeled and minced

1 1/2 teaspoon of minced garlic

2 teaspoons of minced ginger

1 1/2 teaspoon of salt

1/8 teaspoon of ground black pepper

1/4 teaspoon of crushed red pepper

1/4 teaspoon of five spice powder

2 teaspoons of molasses

1 tablespoon of whole-grain mustard

1/4 teaspoon of vegan Worcestershire sauce

8 ounces of tomato sauce

1/4 cup of hoisin sauce

1 tablespoon of soy sauce

2 tablespoons of apple cider vinegar

2 tablespoons of water

Directions:

Take a 6-quarts slow cooker, grease it with a non-stick cooking spray and set it aside until it is required.

Place a medium-sized non-stick skillet pan over an average heat, add the oil and let it heat.

Cut the tofu into 1/2 inch pieces and add it to the skillet pan in a single layer.

Cook for 3 minutes per sides and then transfer it to the prepared slow cooker.

When the tofu turns brown, place it into the pan, add the onion, garlic, ginger and cook for 3 to 5 minutes or until the onions are softened.

Add the remaining ingredients into the pan except for the vegetables which are the broccoli stalks, zucchini, bell pepper and water chestnuts.

Stir until it mixes properly and cook for 2 minutes or until the mixture starts bubbling.

Transfer this mixture into the slow cooker and stir properly.

Cover the top, plug in the slow cooker; adjust the cooking time to 3 hours and let it cook on the high heat setting or until it is cooked thoroughly.

In the meantime, trim the broccoli stalks and cut it into 1/4 inch pieces.

When the tofu is cooked thoroughly, put it into the slow cooker; add the broccoli stalks and the remaining vegetables.

Stir until it mixes properly and then return the top to cover it.

Continue cooking for 1 hour at the high heat setting or until the vegetables are tender.

Serve right away with rice.

Nutrition:

Calories:189 Cal, Carbohydrates:19g, Protein:12g, Fats:9g, Fiber:3g.

Inexpensive Bean and Spinach Enchiladas

Servings: 8

Preparation Time: 3 hours

Ingredients:

2 cups of cooked black beans

1 cup of frozen corn

10 ounce of chopped spinach

Half of a medium-sized cucumber, peeled and sliced

6 cups of chopped lettuce

4 medium-sized radishes, peeled and cut into matchsticks

1/2 cup of cherry tomatoes, halved

1 teaspoon of salt, divided

1/2 teaspoon of ground black pepper, divided

1/2 teaspoon of ground cumin

3 1/2 cups of tomato salsa

2 cups of grated vegetarian cheddar cheese

8 corn tortillas, about 6-inch

3 tablespoons lime juice

2 tablespoons olive oil

Directions:

Place 1 cup of beans in a medium-sized bowl then ,using a fork mash them.

Then add the remaining beans, corn, spinach, 1/2 teaspoon of salt, 1/4 teaspoon of black pepper, 1 cup of cheddar cheese and stir until it mixes well.

Take a 6-quarts slow cooker and spread 2 cups of tomato salsa on the bottom.

Place the tortillas on a clean working space and proportionally top it with the prepared bean mixture, at least 1/2 cup.

Roll up the tortillas and place it into the slow cooker on top of the salsa, seam-side down.

Top it with the remaining tomato salsa, cheese and cover the top.

Plug in the slow cooker; adjust the cooking time to 3 hours and let it cook on the the low heat setting or until the cheese melts completely.

In the meantime, using a bowl, place the cucumber, lettuce, radish and tomatoes in it, sprinkle it with the lime juice, oil, the remaining of each salt and black pepper.

Toss to cover and serve this with the cooked enchiladas.

Nutrition:

Calories:239 Cal, Carbohydrates:31g, Protein:16g, Fats:8.5g, Fiber:9g.

Delightful Coconut Vegetarian Curry

Servings: 6

Preparation Time: 4 hours and 20 minutes

Ingredients:

5 medium-sized potatoes, peeled and cut into 1-inch cubes

1/4 cup of curry powder

2 tablespoons of flour

1 tablespoon of chili powder

1/2 teaspoon of red pepper flakes

1/2 teaspoon of cayenne pepper

1 large green bell pepper, cut into strips

1 large red bell pepper, cut into strips

2 tablespoons of onion soup mix

14-ounce of coconut cream, unsweetened

3 cups of vegetable broth

2 medium-sized carrots, peeled and cut into matchstick

1 cup of green peas

1/4 cup of chopped cilantro

Directions:

Take a 6-quarts slow cooker, grease it with a non-stick cooking spray and place the potatoes pieces in the bottom.

Add the remaining ingredients except for the carrots, peas and cilantro.

Stir properly and cover the top.

Plug in the slow cooker; adjust the cooking time to 4 hours and let it cook on the low heat setting or until it cooks thoroughly.

When the cooking time is over, add the carrots to the curry and continue cooking for 30 minutes.

Then, add the peas and continue cooking for another 30 minutes or until the peas get tender.

Garnish it with cilantro and serve.

Nutrition:

Calories:369 Cal, Carbohydrates:39g, Protein:7g, Fats:23g, Fiber:8g.

Super tasty Vegetarian Chili

Servings: 6

Preparation Time: 2 hours and 10 minutes

Ingredients:

16-ounce of vegetarian baked beans

16 ounce of cooked chickpeas

16 ounce of cooked kidney beans

15 ounce of cooked corn

1 medium-sized green bell pepper, cored and chopped

2 stalks of celery, peeled and chopped

12 ounce of chopped tomatoes

1 medium-sized white onion, peeled and chopped

1 teaspoon of minced garlic

1 teaspoon of salt

1 tablespoon of red chili powder

1 tablespoon of dried oregano

1 tablespoon of dried basil

1 tablespoon of dried parsley

18-ounce of black bean soup

4-ounce of tomato puree

Directions:

Take a 6-quarts slow cooker, grease it with a non-stick cooking spray and place all the ingredients into it.

Stir properly and cover the top.

Plug in the slow cooker; adjust the cooking time to 2 hours and let it cook on the high heat setting or until it is cooked thoroughly.

Serve right away.

Nutrition:

Calories:190 Cal, Carbohydrates:35g, Protein:11g, Fats:1g, Fiber:10g.

Vegetable Soup

Servings: 8

Preparation Time: 6 hours and 30 minutes

Ingredients:

1/4 cup of vegetable shortening

2 cups of all-purpose flour, leveled

1/2 cup of barley, uncooked

16 ounce of diced tomatoes

2 medium-sized potatoes, peeled and cubed

16 ounce of frozen mixed vegetables

1 large white onion, peeled and diced

1 1/2 teaspoon of minced garlic

6 cups of vegetable broth

1/2 teaspoon of salt

1/2 teaspoon of dried basil

1/2 teaspoon of ground black pepper

1 teaspoon of dried oregano

1 teaspoon of dried parsley

1 bay leaf

6 1/4 cup of vegetable broth

Directions:

Take a 6 quarts slow cooker, grease it with a non-stick cooking spray and add all the ingredients except for flour, vegetable shortening and reserve 1/4 cup of vegetable broth.

Stir properly and cover the top.

Plug in the slow cooker; adjust the cooking time to 6 hours and let it cook on the low heat setting or until it is cooked thoroughly.

In the meantime, place the flour, shortening in a food processor and pulse it until the mixture resembles crumbs.

Then gradually mix the reserved 1/4 cup of vegetable broth until the smooth dough comes together.

Transfer the dough to a clean space filled with flour and roll it into the 1/8 thick dough.

Using a sharp knife cut the dough into small squares and put them in the slow cooker when 6 hours of cooking time is over.

Continue cooking for 1 hour at the high heat setting or until the dumplings are soft.

Scoop it into the serving bowls and serve.

Nutrition:

Calories:218 Cal, Carbohydrates:31g, Protein:7g, Fats:8g, Fiber:6g.

Creamy Sweet Potato & Coconut Curry

Servings: 6

Preparation Time: 6 hours and 20 minutes

Ingredients:

2 pounds of sweet potatoes, peeled and chopped

1/2 pound of red cabbage, shredded

2 red chilies, seeded and sliced

2 medium-sized red bell peppers, cored and sliced

2 large white onions, peeled and sliced

1 1/2 teaspoon of minced garlic

1 teaspoon of grated ginger

1/2 teaspoon of salt

1 teaspoon of paprika

1/2 teaspoon of cayenne pepper

2 tablespoons of peanut butter

4 tablespoons of olive oil

12-ounce of tomato puree

14 fluid ounce of coconut milk

1/2 cup of chopped coriander

Directions:

Place a large non-stick skillet pan over an average heat, add 1 tablespoon of oil and let it heat.

Then add the onion and cook for 10 minutes or until it gets soft.

Add the garlic, ginger, salt, paprika, cayenne pepper and continue cooking for 2 minutes or until it starts producing fragrance.

Transfer this mixture to a 6-quarts slow cooker, and reserve the pan.

In the pan, add 1 tablespoon of oil and let it heat.

Add the cabbage, red chili, bell pepper and cook it for 5 minutes.

Then transfer this mixture to the slow cooker and reserve the pan.

Add the remaining oil to the pan; the sweet potatoes in a single layer and cook it in 3 batches for 5 minutes or until it starts getting brown.

Add the sweet potatoes to the slow cooker, along with tomato puree, coconut milk and stir properly.

Cover the top, plug in the slow cooker; adjust the cooking time to 6 hours and let it cook on the low heat setting or until the sweet potatoes are tender.

When done, add the seasoning and pour it in the peanut butter.

Garnish it with coriander and serve.

Nutrition:

Calories:434 Cal, Carbohydrates:47g, Protein:6g, Fats:22g, Fiber:3g.

Comforting Chickpea Tagine

Servings: 6

Preparation Time: 4 hours and 15 minutes

Ingredients:

14 ounce of cooked chickpeas

12 dried apricots

1 red bell pepper, cored and sliced

1 small butternut squash, peeled, cored and chopped

2 zucchini, stemmed and chopped

1 medium-sized white onion, peeled and chopped

1 teaspoon of minced garlic

1 teaspoon of ground ginger

1 1/2 teaspoon of salt

1 teaspoon of ground black pepper

1 teaspoon of ground cumin

2 teaspoon of paprika

1 teaspoon of harissa paste

2 teaspoon of honey

2 tablespoons of olive oil

1 pound of passata

1/4 cup of chopped coriander

Directions:

Take a 6-quarts slow cooker, grease it with a non-stick cooking spray and place the chickpeas, apricots, bell pepper, butternut squash, zucchini and onion into it.

Sprinkle it with salt, black pepper and set it aside until it is called for.

Place a large non-stick skillet pan over an average temperature of heat; add the oil, garlic, cumin and paprika.

Stir properly and cook for 1 minutes or until it starts producing fragrance.

Then pour in the harissa paste, honey, passata and boil the mixture.

When the mixture is done boiling, pour this mixture over the vegetables in the slow cooker and cover it with the lid.

Plug in the slow cooker; adjust the cooking time to 4 hours and let it cook on the high heat setting or until the vegetables gets tender.

When done, add the seasoning, garnish it with the coriander and serve right away.

Nutrition:

Calories:237 Cal, Carbohydrates:45g, Protein:9g, Fats:2g, Fiber:8g.

Curried Tofu

Preparation Time: 30 mins.

Servings: 4

Nutrition: Calories: 345, Carbohydrates: 37 g, Proteins: 33.9 g, Fats: 6.3 g

Ingredients:

¼ t. garlic powder

2 tbsp. curry powder

1 pack extra firm tofu

Directions:

Heat to 400 degrees the oven.

Slice the tofu into cubes.

In a container with a lid, add the garlic powder, curry powder, and cubed tofu.

Close it tightly and shake lightly just to coat the tofu. Make sure there's even coverage of the spices.

On a parchment-lined cookie sheet, place the tofu cubes and bake for 15 minutes, flip and continue baking for another 15 minutes or until crisp.

Serve warm and enjoy!

Sesame Tofu and Eggplant

Preparation Time: 20 mins.

Servings: 4

Nutrition: Calories: 295, Carbohydrates: 6.87 g, Proteins: 11.21 g, Fats: 6.87 g

Ingredients:

1 tbsp. olive oil

¼ c. of the following:

sesame seeds

soy sauce

1 eggplant

1 pound firm tofu

1 t. crushed red pepper flakes

2 cloves garlic

2 t. sweetener of your choice

4 tbsp. toasted sesame oil

1 c. cilantro, chopped

3 tbsp. rice vinegar

Salt and pepper to taste

Directions:

Set the oven to 200 heat setting.

Remove the tofu from the package and blot using paper towels to absorb excess moisture.

In a big mixing bowl, whisk together red pepper flakes, garlic, sesame oil, vinegar, and ¼ cup of cilantro to create the marinade.

With a mandolin, julienne the eggplant. If you do not have this, you can create the noodles by hand.

Mix the noodles in the big bowl with the marinade.

Add oil to a skillet over medium-low flame setting, and cook the eggplant until soft.

Turn off the oven, and add the last of the cilantro.

Transfer the contents from the skillet to an oven-safe dish, cover with foil, and place in the oven to keep warm.

Cut the tofu into 8 slices and coat with sesame seeds. Press the sesame seeds into the tofu.

In the skillet, add 2 tablespoons of sesame oil and warm under medium heat. Fry the tofu for five minutes then flip and fry.

Pour the soy sauce into the pan, coating the tofu. Cook until the tofu looks caramelized.

Remove the noodles from the oven and plate with the tofu on top of the noodles.

Serve warm and enjoy!

Tempeh Coconut Curry

Preparation Time: 30 mins.

Servings: 4

Nutrition: Calories: 558, Carbohydrates: 54.2 g, Proteins: 18.4 g, Fats: 33.5 g

Curry:

2 t. of the following:

low-sodium soy sauce

tamarind pulp

1 tbsp. of the following:

lime juice

garlic, finely chopped

ginger, finely chopped

vegetable oil

salt

8 oz. tempeh

13.5 oz. coconut milk, light

1 c. water

3 c. sweet potato, chopped

1 cinnamon stick

½ t. of the following:

red pepper, crushed

turmeric, ground

1 ½ t. coriander, ground

2 c. onion, finely chopped

Rice:

1 ½ c. cauliflower rice

¼ t. salt

1/3 c. cilantro, chopped

Directions:

Using a medium-high heat setting, warm some oil in a big pot or whatever you prefer, as long as it's nonstick.

Place the onion and ½ teaspoon of salt and sauté for approximately 2 minutes.

Next, stir in the tamarind, breaking it up as you combine in the skillet and cooking for another 2 minutes.

Add in the ginger, garlic, coriander, turmeric, crushed red pepper, and cinnamon stick; stir constantly.

Add in the additional salt, tempeh, milk, water, and potatoes, bringing to a boil.

Cover, allowing to simmer for fifteen minutes or until tender.

Whisk in the soy sauce and simmer for 3 additional minutes.

Remove the cinnamon stick.

Cook the cauliflower rice according to package instructions.

Stir in the cilantro.

Place the rice in a bowl and cover with curry.
Serve warm and enjoy!

Tempeh Tikka Masala

Preparation Time: 1 h, 35 mins.

Servings: 3

Nutrition: Calories: 430, Carbohydrates: 39 g,
Proteins: 21 g, Fats: 23 g

Tempeh:

½ t. sea salt

1 t. of the following:

gram masala

ginger, ground

cumin, ground

2 t. apple cider vinegar

½ c. vegan yogurt

8 oz. tempeh, cubed

Tikka Masala Sauce:

2 c. frozen peas

1 c. of the following:

full-fat coconut milk

tomato sauce

¼ t. turmeric

½ t. sea salt

1 onion, chopped

1 t. of the following:

chili powder

garam masala

1/4 c. ginger, freshly grated

3 cloves garlic, minced

1 tbsp. coconut oil

Directions:

Begin with making the tempeh by combining sea salt, garam masala, ginger, cumin, vinegar, and yogurt in a bowl.

Add tempeh to the bowl and coat well; cover the bowl and refrigerate for 60 minutes.

In a pan big enough for 3 servings, add some coconut oil to heat using the medium setting, and begin preparing the sauce.

Sauté in the ginger, garlic, and onion for 5 minutes or until fragrant.

Add the garam masala, chili powder, sea salt, and turmeric and combine well.

Add the frozen peas, coconut, milk, tomato sauce, and tempeh, reducing the heat to medium.

Simmer for 15 minutes

Caprice Casserole

Preparation Time: 1 h, 35 mins.

Servings: 3

Nutrition: Calories: 642, Carbohydrates: 88.6 g, Proteins: 25.1 g, Fats: 5.1 g

Tempeh:

¼ c. basil, chopped

1 tomato, big

¼ t. pepper

½ t. salt

1 tbsp. of the following:

nutritional yeast

tahini

1 clove garlic

14 oz. tofu, extra firm, drained

6 cups marinara sauce

10 oz. vegetable noodles

Directions:

Set the oven to 350 heat setting.

Cut the tofu into 4 slabs and remove excess moisture by gently squeezing each slab with a paper towel.

In a food processor, add garlic and chop, then scrape garlic from the sides to ensure it will be thoroughly mixed.

Add pepper, salt, yeast, tahini, and tofu to the food processor and pulse for 15 to 20 seconds until fully combined and forming a paste.

In an oven-safe dish, spread ½ cup of the marinara sauce across the bottom.

Divide the vegetable noodles in half, break the noodles, and layer them on top of the sauce.

Add another layer of sauce on top of the noodles.

Add the remaining noodles and coat the top with remaining sauce.

Using the tofu mixture from the food processor, form little patties about ½ thick and place on top of the sauce, filling up the dish.

Cover the baking container with aluminum foil and bake for 20 minutes.

Uncover and bake for an additional fifteen minutes.

Remove from the oven and set the oven to broil.

Place the tomato slices on top of tofu mixture and broil for 2 minutes or until the tofu is lightly toasted.

Garnish with basil.

Serve warm and enjoy.

Cheesy Brussel Sprout Bake

Preparation Time: 45 mins.

Servings: 8

Nutrition: Calories: 116, Carbohydrates: 16 g, Proteins: 4 g, Fats: 4 g

Ingredients:

½ onion sliced

2 tbsp. of each of these

garlic, chopped

avocado oil

1 ½ lb. Brussel sprouts

Cheese:

Dash cayenne

1 t. of the following:

onion powder

salt

¼ t. of the following:

pepper

paprika

½ t. of the following:

garlic, powder

thyme

1 tbsp. tapioca starch

¼ c. nutritional yeast

½ c. vegetable broth

1 can coconut cream

Crumble Topping :

¼ t. pepper

½ t. garlic, powder

1 t. salt

½ c. panko crumbs

Directions:

Bring the oven to 425 heat setting.

Prepare Brussel sprouts by washing and trimming then steaming for 10 minutes.

Spray an oven-safe baking dish with nonstick spray.

Add the Brussel sprouts to a baking dish and set to the side.

Bring a skillet to medium temperature and mix in the garlic, avocado oil, and onion, sautéing approximately 6 minutes.

Add the onion mixture to the top of the Brussel sprouts.

In the same skillet on low heat, add vegetable broth, nutritional yeast, onion powder, pepper, salt, garlic, paprika, thyme, and coconut cream, whisking together to combine.

Carefully add in the tapioca starch and whisk constantly; the mixture will thicken in about 5 minutes.

Once it turns into a cheese sauce mixture, pour over the Brussel sprouts and onions.

In a mixing container, combine panko, salt, garlic, and pepper, creating the crumble.

Sprinkle the crumble across the top of the cheese.

Cook in the oven for approximately 25 minutes or until browned and golden.

Serve warm and enjoy.

Tofu Noodle Bowl

Preparation Time: 45 mins.

Servings: 4

Nutrition: Calories: 669, Carbohydrates: 69 g, Proteins: 55.1 g, Fats: 24.7g

Ingredients:

¼ c. of the following

peanuts, chopped

cilantro, chopped

4 heads baby bok choy, chopped

2 packages premade baked tofu, 8 oz.

½ t. black pepper, ground

2 t. of the following:

turmeric, ground

garlic chili sauce

1 tbsp. of the following:

lime juice

ginger, minced

2 c. vegetable stock

2 carrots, julienned

1 red bell pepper, chopped

½ red onion, diced

2 cloves garlic, minced

1 t. peanut oil

6 oz. Thai rice noodles

Directions:

Prepare the Thai noodles, following the package guidelines or according to your preference.

Warm a big pan using medium-high heat, adding in the peanut oil.

Sauté the ginger, garlic, and onion for approximately 5 minutes.

Next, add in the carrots and bell pepper, stirring frequently and cooking for 5 minutes.

Whisk together the lime juice, black pepper, turmeric, chili sauce, and stock, then combine with the pan of peppers and carrots.

Wait for the mixture to boil, and soon after, bring down the heat setting, and leave it cooking for nearly 5 minutes.

As it simmers, add in the noodles, bok choy, and tofu and cook for an additional 5 minutes.

Divide between bowls and garnish with chili peppers, peanuts, and cilantro.

Serve warm and enjoy.

Cashew Siam Salad

Preparation Time: 25 mins.

Servings: 4

Nutrition: Calories: 352, Carbohydrates: 26.6 g, Proteins: 9.6 g, Fats: 24.5 g

Ingredients:

3 green onions, chopped

2/3 c. sunflower seeds

1 bag slaw mix

2 packages ramen noodles

1 c. cashews, crushed

1 t. olive oil

Dressing:

Seasoning packets from ramen noodles

1 c. vinegar

½ c. sweetener of your choice

Directions:

Set the oven to 350 heat setting.

In a mixing container, combine cashews and oil and mix until the nuts are lightly oiled.

Place the nuts on a lined cookie sheet and toast until lightly browned in the oven.

In a big mixing bowl, crumble the ramen noodles and combine with slaw mix, sunflower seeds, and green onion.

Whisk together the vinegar and sweetener of your choice in a little bowl until combined.

Remove the peanuts from the oven and cool.

Place the salad in a bowl and cover the top with peanuts.

When ready to serve, add the dressing, and enjoy.

Cucumber Edamame Salad

Preparation Time: 2 hours mins.

Servings: 8

Nutrition: Calories: 166, Carbohydrates: 6.4 g, Proteins: 2.9 g, Fats: 14.9 g

Ingredients:

1 jalapeno pepper, seeded and chopped

2 c. froze edamame, shelled and thawed

4 English cucumbers, spiralizer

Vinaigrette:

1 t. red pepper flakes

1 ½ t. of the following:

garlic

Dijon mustard

soy sauce, low-sodium

2 t. ginger, paste

3 t. toasted sesame oil

1/3 c. of the following:

rice vinegar

extra virgin olive oil

Directions:

Begin by cleaning your cucumbers and spiraling them to create the noodles.

Once cucumbers are spiraled, use a towel or cheesecloth to discard the excess moisture out of the noodles.

In a big mixing bowl, add noodles, jalapeno, red bell pepper, and edamame. Carefully toss the salad mixture and set to the side.

In a little mixing container, prepare the vinaigrette by whisking together the red pepper flakes, garlic, Dejon, soy sauce, ginger, oil, rice vinegar, and olive oil.

Lightly coat the salad with dressing.

Cover and refrigerate overnight or a minimum of 2 hours.

Serve cool and enjoy.

Caesar Vegan Salad

Preparation Time: 30 mins.

Servings: 6

Nutrition: Calories: 284, Carbohydrates: 25.5 g, Proteins: 8.7 g, Fats: 18.4 g

Ingredients:

5 c. kale, chopped

10 c. romaine lettuce

Cheese:

½ t. garlic

1 tbsp. of the following:

extra virgin olive oil

nutritional yeast

1 garlic clove

2 tbsp. hemp seeds, hulled

1/3 c. cashews, raw

Caesar Dressing:

½ t. of the following:

sea salt

garlic powder

Dijon mustard

2 t. capers

½ tbsp. vegan Worcestershire sauce

2 tbsp. olive oil (best if extra virgin)

½ c. raw cashews, soaked overnight

¼ c. water

1 clove garlic, crushed

1 tbsp. lemon juice

Croutons:

1/8 t. cayenne pepper

½ t. of the following:

garlic powder

sea salt

1 t. olive oil, (best if extra virgin)

14 oz. can chickpeas

Directions:

On the day before you plan to make this salad, in a little bowl, soak ½ c. of the raw cashews overnight then drain and rinse.

For the Croutons – Bring the oven to 400 heat setting. Drain the chickpeas and rinse thoroughly. Using a tea towel or cheesecloth, rub the chickpeas so that the skins fall off. Place those in a dish for baking. Spritz the chickpeas with oil and roll them around to coat. Season with cayenne, salt, and garlic powder. Roast the chickpeas for approximately a quarter of an hour or until you are satisfied with the color. Remove from the oven, allowing to cool and become firm.

For the Dressing – Combine everything but not the salt, either in a processor or blender. Blend until smooth liquid consistency. If needed, add ½ tablespoon of water at a time until you have a dressing-like consistency. Season with salt to taste. Set to the side.

For the Cheese – In a food processor, add garlic and cashews and process them until they reach a finely chopped consistency. Add hemp seeds, nutritional yeast, olive oil, and garlic powder and blend until combined. Season with salt to taste.

For the lettuce – After washing the kale, finely chop and set to the side. Chop the lettuce roughly into 2-inch pieces and toss with the kale in a bowl.

Pour some dressing and toss again to coat the greens fully.

Sprinkle the cheese and croutons over the top.

Serve cool and enjoy.

Mushroom Lettuce Wraps

Preparation Time: 30 mins.

Servings: 4

Nutrition: Calories: 265, Carbohydrates: 37.6 g, Proteins: 13.6 g, Fats: 7.9 g

Ingredients:

8 big leaf romaine lettuce

4 green onions, sliced

¼ t. red pepper flakes

2 t. of the following:

ginger, grated

canola oil

2 cloves garlic

12 oz. extra firm tofu

1 t. sesame oil

2 tbsp. rice vinegar

8 oz. mushrooms, diced

1 can water chestnuts

3 tbsp. of the following:

soy sauce, reduced-sodium

hoisin Sauce

Directions:

Whisk together in a little bowl the sesame oil, rice vinegar, soy sauce, and hoisin. Then set to the side.

Open the tofu, and using a paper towel or cheesecloth, remove as much liquid as you can.

In a big skillet over medium-high heat, warm the 2 teaspoons of canola oil.

Crumble the tofu, making it into little pieces and cook for approximately 5 minutes.

Add in the diced mushrooms and cook until almost all the liquid evaporates.

Add in the green onions, red pepper, ginger, garlic, and chestnuts and cook for about 30 seconds.

Pour the sauce from the little bowl into the skillet and cook until sauce is thoroughly warmed.

Plate the individual lettuce leaves and spoon the tofu mixture into each lettuce wrap.

Serve and enjoy warm.

Chapter 10. Smoothies

Chocolate pb smoothie

Preparation time: 5 minutes

Cooking Time: 0 minutes

Servings: 4

Ingredients

1 banana

¼ Cup rolled oats, or 1 scoop plant protein powder

1 tablespoon flaxseed, or chia seeds

1 tablespoon unsweetened cocoa powder

1 tablespoon peanut butter, or almond or sunflower seed butter

1 tablespoon maple syrup (optional)

1 cup alfalfa sprouts, or spinach, chopped (optional)

½ Cup non-dairy milk (optional)

1 cup water

Optional

1 teaspoon maca powder

1 teaspoon cocoa nibs

Directions

Purée everything in a blender until smooth, adding more water (or non-dairy milk) if needed. Add bonus boosters, as desired. Purée until blended.

Nutrition: calories: 474; protein: 13g; total fat: 16g; carbohydrates: 79g; fiber: 18g

Berry beetsicle smoothie

Preparation time: 3 minutes

Cooking Time: 0minutes

Servings: 1

Ingredients

½ Cup peeled and diced beets

½ Cup frozen raspberries

1 frozen banana

1 tablespoon maple syrup

1 cup unsweetened soy or almond milk

Directions

Combine all the ingredients in a blender and blend until smooth.

Green breakfast smoothie

Preparation time: 10 minutes

Cooking Time: 0 minutes

Servings: 2

Ingredients

½ Banana, sliced

2 cups spinach or other greens, such as kale

1 cup sliced berries of your choosing, fresh or frozen

1 orange, peeled and cut into segments

1 cup unsweetened nondairy milk

1 cup ice

Directions

In a blender, combine all the ingredients.

Starting with the blender on low speed, begin blending the smoothie, gradually increasing blender speed until smooth. Serve immediately.

Blueberry lemonade smoothie

Preparation time: 5 minutes

Cooking Time: 0 minutes

Servings: 1

Ingredients

1 cup roughly chopped kale

¾ Cup frozen blueberries

1 cup unsweetened soy or almond milk

Juice of 1 lemon

1 tablespoon maple syrup

Directions

Combine all the ingredients in a blender and blend until smooth. Enjoy immediately.

Berry protein smoothie

Preparation time: 5 minutes

Cooking Time: 0 minutes

Servings: 1

Ingredients

1 banana

1 cup fresh or frozen berries

¾ Cup water or nondairy milk, plus more as needed

1 scoop plant-based protein powder, 3 ounces silken tofu, ¼ cup rolled oats, or ½ cup cooked quinoa

Additions

 1 tablespoon ground flaxseed or chia seeds

 1 handful fresh spinach or lettuce, or 1 chunk cucumber

Coconut water to replace some of the liquid

Directions

Preparing the ingredients

In a blender, combine the banana, berries, water, and your choice of protein.

Add any addition ingredients as desired. Purée until smooth and creamy, about 50 seconds.

Add a bit more water if you like a thinner smoothie.

Nutrition: calories: 332; protein: 7g; total fat: 5g; saturated fat: 1g; carbohydrates: 72g; fiber: 11g

Blueberry and chia smoothie

Preparation time: 10 minutes

Cooking Time: 0 minutes

Servings: 2

Ingredients

2 tablespoons chia seeds

2 cups unsweetened nondairy milk

2 cups blueberries, fresh or frozen

2 tablespoons pure maple syrup or agave

2 tablespoons cocoa powder

Directions

Preparing the ingredients

Soak the chia seeds in the almond milk for 5 minutes. In a blender, combine the soaked chia seeds, almond milk, blueberries, maple syrup, and cocoa powder and blend until smooth. Serve immediately.

Green kickstart smoothie

Preparation time: 5 minutes

Cooking Time: 0 minutes

Servings: 1

Ingredients

½ Avocado or 1 banana

½ Cup chopped cucumber, peeled if desired

1 handful fresh spinach or chopped lettuce

1 pear or apple, peeled and cored, or 1 cup unsweetened applesauce

2 tablespoons freshly squeezed lime juice

1 cup water or nondairy milk, plus more as needed

Additions

½-Inch piece peeled fresh ginger

1 tablespoon ground flaxseed or chia seeds

½ Cup soy yogurt or 3 ounces silken tofu

Coconut water to replace some of the liquid

2 tablespoons chopped fresh mint or ½ cup chopped mango

Directions

Preparing the ingredients

In a blender, combine the avocado, cucumber, spinach, pear, lime juice, and water.

Add any additions ingredients as desired. Purée until smooth and creamy, about 50 seconds. Add a bit more water if you like a thinner smoothie.

Nutrition: calories: 263; protein: 4g; total fat: 14g; saturated fat: 2g; carbohydrates: 36g; fiber: 10g

Chocolate Smoothie

Preparation Time: 5 min.

Servings: 2

Nutrition: Calories: 147, Carbohydrates: 8.2 g, Proteins: 4 g, Fats: 13.4 g

Ingredients:

¼ c. almond butter

¼ c. cocoa powder, unsweetened

½ c. coconut milk, canned

1 c. almond milk, unsweetened

Directions:

Before making the smoothie, freeze the almond milk into cubes using an ice cube tray. This would take a few hours, so prepare it ahead.

Blend everything using your preferred machine until it reaches your desired thickness.

Serve immediately and enjoy!

Chocolate Mint Smoothie

Preparation Time: 5 min.

Servings: 1

Nutrition: Calories: 401, Carbohydrates: 6.3 g, Proteins: 5 g, Fats: 40.3 g

Ingredients:

2 tbsp. sweetener of your choice

2 drops mint extract

1 tbsp. cocoa powder

½ avocado, medium

¼ c. coconut milk

1 c. almond milk, unsweetened

Directions:

In a high-speed blender, add all the ingredients and blend until smooth.

Add two to four ice cubes and blend.

Cinnamon Roll Smoothie

Preparation Time: 2 min.

Servings: 1

Nutrition: Calories: 507, Carbohydrates: 17 g, Proteins: 33.3 g, Fats: 34.9 g

Ingredients:

1 t. cinnamon

1 scoop vanilla protein powder

½ c. of the following:

almond milk, unsweetened

coconut milk

Sweetener of your choice

Directions:

In a high-speed blender, add all the ingredients and blend.

Add two to four ice cubes and blend until smooth.

Serve immediately and enjoy!

Coconut Smoothie

Preparation Time: 2 min.

Servings: 2

Nutrition: Calories: 584, Carbohydrates: 22.5 g, Proteins: 8.3 g, Fats: 55.5 g

Ingredients:

1 t. chia seeds

1/8 c. almonds, soaked

1 c. coconut milk

1 avocado

Directions:

In a high-speed blender, add all the ingredients and blend until smooth.

Add your desired number of ice cubes, depending on your favored consistency, of course, and blend again.

Serve immediately and enjoy!

Maca Almond Smoothie

Preparation Time: 5 min.

Servings: 2

Nutrition: Calories: 758, Carbohydrates: 28.6 g, Proteins: 9.3 g, Fats: 72.3 g

Ingredients:

½ t. vanilla extract

1 scoop maca powder

1 tbsp. almond butter

1 c. almond milk, unsweetened

2 avocados

Directions:

In a high-speed blender, add all the ingredients and blend until smooth.

Serve immediately and enjoy!

Blueberry Smoothie

Preparation Time: 5 min.

Servings: 1

Nutrition: Calories: 401, Carbohydrates: 6.3 g, Proteins: 5 g, Fats: 40.3 g

Ingredients:

¼ c. pumpkin seeds shelled unsalted

3 c. blueberries, frozen

2 avocados, peeled and halved

1 c. almond milk

Directions:

In a high-speed blender, add all the ingredients and blend until smooth.

Add two to four ice cubes and blend until smooth.

Serve immediately and enjoy!

Nutty Protein Shake

Preparation Time: 5 min.

Servings: 1

Nutrition: Calories: 694, Carbohydrates: 30.8 g, Proteins: 40.8 g, Fats: 52 g

Ingredients:

¼ avocado

2 tbsp. powdered peanut butter

1 tbsp. of the following:

Cocoa powder

Peanut butter

1 scoop protein powder

½ c. almond milk

Directions:

In a high-speed blender, add all the ingredients and blend until smooth.

Add two to four ice cubes and blend again.

Serve immediately and enjoy!

Cinnamon Pear Smoothie

Preparation Time: 2 min.

Servings: 1

Nutrition: Calories: 653, Carbohydrates: 75.2 g, Proteins: 28.4 g, Fats: 32.2 g

Ingredients:

1 t. cinnamon

1 scoop vanilla protein powder

½ c. of the following:

Almond milk, unsweetened

Coconut Milk

2 pears, cores removed

Sweetener of your choice

Directions:

In a high-speed blender, add all the ingredients and blend.

Add two or more ice cubes and blend again.

Serve immediately and enjoy!

Vanilla Milkshake

Preparation Time: 5 min.

Servings: 4

Nutrition: Calories: 125, Carbohydrates: 6.8 g, Proteins: 1.2 g, Fats: 11.5 g

Ingredients:

2 c. ice cubes

2 t. vanilla extract

6 tbsp. powdered erythritol

1 c. cream of dairy-free

½ c. coconut milk

Directions:

In a high-speed blender, add all the ingredients and blend.

Add ice cubes and blend until smooth.

Serve immediately and enjoy!

Raspberry Protein Shake

Preparation Time: 5 min.

Servings: 1

Nutrition: Calories: 756, Carbohydrates: 80.1 g, Proteins: 27.6 g, Fats: 40.7 g

Ingredients:

¼ avocado

1 c. raspberries, frozen

1 scoop protein powder

½ c. almond milk

Ice cubes

Directions:

In a high-speed blender add all the ingredients and blend until lumps of fruit disappear.

Add two to four ice cubes and blend to your desired consistency.

Serve immediately and enjoy!

Raspberry Almond Smoothie

Preparation Time: 5 min.

Servings: 1

Nutrition: Calories: 449, Carbohydrates: 26 g, Proteins: 14 g, Fats: 35 g

Ingredients:

10 Almonds, finely chopped

3 tbsp. almond butter

1 c. almond milk

1 c. Raspberries, frozen

Directions:

In a high-speed blender, add all the ingredients and blend until smooth.

Serve immediately and enjoy!

Chapter 11. Cooking Tips

If you are concerned about the affordability of being vegan, don't despair, as there are many tips and tricks for cheaper eating.

Learn to Make a Couple of Great Pot Meals:

Chilies, curries and other pot meals can be a fantastic way to stretch out your food budget. Most pot meals can be paired with rice or other inexpensive grains to make a satisfying yet cheap lunch or dinner. While making a large pot meal can take a little more time initially, you can save time later in the week, as all you need to do is reheat.

Prepare Your Own Lunches:

Another money saving tip that applies to vegans and non-vegans alike is to prepare your own lunches. While spending a couple of dollars on a sandwich for lunch may not seem like much, when you add in buying a drink, chips and something sweet for dessert, you could be spending hundreds of dollars a month. It will cost only a fraction of this to buy in the ingredients to make your own lunches, saving you a small fortune over the course of a year. If you are taking your lunch to school or work, you can get a little more creative than just a dull sandwich. Why not pack a colorful bean salad? Or take a container of your leftover curry and rice to be heated in the break room? There are so many tasty vegan lunch ideas that you can enjoy a delicious meal and save money.

Plan Your Meals and Grocery Shopping:

We've all done it. Grocery shopping when we have no idea what we're going to cook will end up with all sorts of things in our cart. Impulse buying ingredients is likely to mean that when you do get home, you won't have all you need for full meals. However, by planning out what meals you plan on making this week and following a shopping list, you can keep the cost of your groceries lower. You will also find that you are less likely to impulse buy costly snacks or premade foods. Be sure to have a healthy vegan snack before you go grocery shopping to keep those sugar-laden treats out of your shopping cart.

Conclusion

If you want to live a healthier and happier life, take the first step towards good nutrition.

Start with a diet like plant-based diet program, which has been proven in scientific research to be beneficial to health, but at the same time, is not too strict and stringent.

Follow the recipes and techniques presented in this book to achieve the best results.

Good luck!